Simplified Nutrition and Weight Management

from the Perpetual Student

Twelve years of dietetic courses and subsequent nutrition registrations
condensed into one, easy-to-understand guidebook!

Shannon Deshazer, NDTR, CDM

The information presented in this book is compiled from sources considered to be reliable and represent the best professional judgment in the nutrition field. The author makes no representations or warranties in regards to accuracy or completeness of the contents within this book. Information used in this book is at the reader's discretion and a health care professional should always be consulted in regards to the reader's specific situation. The accuracy of the information is not guaranteed, nor is any responsibility assumed or implied by the author or publisher.

F&N Publishing

ISBN-13: 978-1543137415
ISBN-10: 1543137415

Printed in the United States of America

Dedicated to

My beautiful husband of sixteen years, Jason, for sticking by me even when he's seen me at my worst. My all and my everything at the end of the day: my faith and my sweet children.

Acknowledgements

I would like to start out by thanking my mom, Renae Bolden, for being a great role model for higher education, proofing my work and always being biased in my favor. Cary Deshazer has done a great job allowing me to add more proofreading to her already editing-full life and being patient with my many, many changes. I am thankful my husband, Jason Deshazer, took time out of his busy schedule to digitize my chemical structures. Thank you to Diana Boos for freely sharing your recipes with me. I would like to thank Shannon McMahon, MS, RD, LD, my professor and advisor, who has been a great help through my school years and continues to be a source of encouragement. Teressa Wray RDN, LDN, always patient and kind with me through my internship period, and even now, and I am grateful for that. Sharon Judy, RN, was a great help utilizing her science and research background to review my work. I would also like to thank Dustin Hawkins for letting me pick his brain about publishing. Who can forget the dads? Thank you to my dad, Dennis Bolden, for being an avid reader and passing on your love of reading to me, which, in turn, became a love of writing. Thank you to Jeff Deshazer for being a great example of strong work ethic.

Photo credits

Me for being an awesome photographer (haha), Huntsville, AL for being so photography-worthy and my family for being "willing" participants.

About the Author

Shannon Deshazer is a wife, mother of a 7-year-old daughter, 7-month old boy and a perpetual student. She and her husband moved all over the country during his active military days and military contracting work. As a result, she has attended 7 different colleges and has taken over 150 credits equaling about 61 classes; 34 of those are related to nutrition. Take it from her: she's learned a thing or two about nutrition.

Her passion is nutrition and weight counseling, utilizing weight management techniques of a healthy, yet balanced, lifestyle for long-term results. Through this long schooling process, she always tried her best to jot down the most pertinent information in order to potentially help others. As a Nutrition and Dietetics Technician, Registered, Shannon is able to discuss nutrition and prevention with healthy individuals. She cannot treat, and will not treat, any nutrition-related diseases. This book is entirely focused on helping to achieve and maintain a healthy weight and a healthy lifestyle.

So whether you are a perpetual student, like Shannon, and your objective is to help others reach their personal goals OR you have been on a perpetual hunt for motivation to begin, persist, reach, maintain and CELEBRATE your quest for healthy living, she hopes this book meets you where you are and can take you on that life-long pursuit – living happy, healthy and well informed.

Contents

Chapter 1

Caloric Intake and Balanced Eating Tips Overview

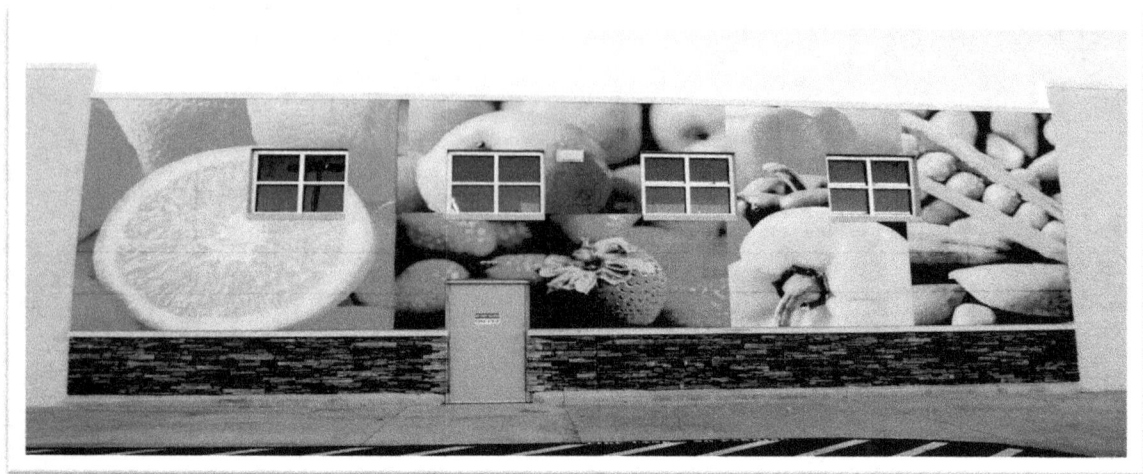

Note: Before you get too comfortable, please grab a pencil (and paper if you prefer not to write in the book). You might also want to keep a basic calculator nearby if you prefer calculations over tables. In chapter 2, you will need a calculator and measuring tape.

We're going to start off slow, with concepts you might have covered before. Our goal during this time is to raise awareness of different food and lifestyle habits in your life. A few chapters later, we'll move into the counseling portion where we'll work toward making positive changes for any nutrition and weight loss goals you might have.

I also want you to be able to benefit from my hours and hours (and more hours) of class time, so I'll share with you the science behind nutrition. Don't worry; I'll try not to weigh it down too much. I'll try to provide just enough for you to have some good take-away information.

Finally, we'll wrap it up with some follow-up counseling. I want you to be able to come back to this book time and time again for help with goal setting and to even learn more about some of the science behind particular goals you may eventually want to work toward.

I ask that you let nutrition and lifestyle change become positive words in your life. Take your time with this book and this process. Good nutrition, and thus lasting positive effects, is an on-going experience. Allow yourself time to really let the information sink in. Allow yourself to work toward positive goals in your life. You'll thank yourself in the long run.

Okay. So, without further ado, let's begin!

Let's start off with some great exercises to help bring awareness (and eventual change) to your life.

Walk me through your day. Write down any and all food and drinks you consumed on a typical day (say, yesterday) from the time you woke up to the time you went to bed.

_____   _____   _____

_____   _____   _____

_____   _____   _____

_____   _____   _____

_____   _____   _____

_____   _____   _____

_____   _____   _____

_____   _____   _____

_____   _____   _____

_____   _____   _____

_____   _____   _____

Okay, let's take a look at serving sizes.

Serving Size Chart

FOOD	HAND-SIZE COMPARISON	SERVING SIZE
Grains		
Dry cereal	One fist	1 cup
Noodles, rice, oatmeal	Handful	½ cup
Whole wheat bread	Flat hand	1 slice
Vegetables		
Cooked vegetable	One fist	1 cup
Salad	Two fists	2 cups
Fruits		
Whole fruit	One fist	1 medium fruit
Canned fruit	One fist	1 cup
Dairy		
Milk and yogurt	One fist	1 cup
Cheese	Index finger	1 ½ ounces
Protein		
Chicken, beef, fish, pork	Palm size	3 ounces
Peanut butter	Thumb	1 tablespoon

Table 1: Adapted from: Dairy Council of California

1. Please go back through your 24-hour recall list and try your best to describe the serving sizes using the chart provided on the previous page. Mark down how many servings you had of that item next to your original list.
2. Go ahead and write down your servings of fluids as well because we'll be using that in a later section. You can use 1 fist size = 1 cup as a reference if you need.

Did you try and compare your serving sizes to the chart? How did you do? Did you find that you are eating more than the recommended serving sizes in one sitting?

*Helpful hint: Pile on the vegetables at dinner. They are filling, which can keep second helpings to a minimum.

Let's add in food groups. We all remember learning about the U.S. Department of Agriculture (USDA) MyPyramid, but now it has been updated to MyPlate. This update includes changing over to cup and ounce equivalents to determine serving sizes. It sounds intimidating, but you'll get the hang of it. You've already listed what you had to eat and drink yesterday, as well as the approximate equivalent size.

3. Now go through each item on your list and put a check mark in the boxes below for each serving of grain, vegetable, fruit, protein and dairy.
4. If you had any dessert, sugary drinks or other empty calories just include that at the bottom.

As always, be honest because you can't help yourself if you're busy sabotaging yourself!

Grains:

Vegetables:

Fruits:

Protein:

Dairy:

NOT a food group, but important to list:

Dessert:

_____

Sugary drinks:

_____

Other empty calories:

_____

How did you do? Were you missing any food groups entirely? Did you find that you had 0 of one thing and 8 or so of another? If so, no big deal, we'll work on that.

At this point, you might be thinking, "Lady, my weight loss goals are bigger than an apple. Why are you asking these questions?" Well, I have good reason to be asking. If you are really low in food group areas or really high in serving sizes of foods, then that is a sign of two potential red flags that we might want to work on:

1. You are missing out on important nutrients that come with eating a variety of healthy foods
2. You might be filling the food group voids with foods that are higher in fat and higher in calories (and thus eventual weight gain).

Here's a piece of fun information!

Place a large mirror in front of where you eat. For example, in the kitchen, living room or dining room!

A Cornell University study showed that eating unhealthy foods in front of a mirror made the food taste less appetizing, which led to less eating of that unhealthy food.[1]

Alright, let's determine how many calories you need each day. This will help us when discussing how much food you are taking in versus what is needed. A chart is provided to help you determine caloric needs based on sex, age and activity level:

5. Find and circle (or write down) your calories in the next chart so you can have a quick reference.

Daily Caloric Intake Needs

Activity Level Age	MALE			FEMALE		
	Sedentary	Moderately Active	Active	Sedentary	Moderately Active	Active
2	1,000	1000	1000	1000	1000	1000
3	1200	1400	1400	1000	1200	1400
4	1200	1400	1600	1200	1400	1400
5	1200	1400	1600	1200	1400	1600
6	1400	1600	1800	1200	1400	1600
7	1400	1600	1800	1200	1600	1800
8	1400	1600	2000	1400	1600	1800
9	1600	1800	2000	1400	1600	1800
10	1600	1800	2200	1400	1800	2000
11	1800	2000	2200	1600	1800	2000
12	1800	2200	2400	1600	2000	2200
13	2000	2200	2600	1600	2000	2200
14	2000	2400	2800	1800	2000	2400
15	2200	2600	3000	1800	2000	2400
16	2400	2800	3200	1800	2000	2400
17	2400	2800	3200	1800	2000	2400
18	2400	2800	3200	1800	2000	2400
19-20	2600	2800	3000	2000	2200	2400
21-25	2400	2800	3000	2000	2000	2400
26-30	2400	2600	3000	1800	2000	2400
31-35	2400	2600	3000	1800	2000	2200
36-40	2400	2600	2800	1800	2000	2200
41-45	2200	2600	2800	1800	2000	2200
46-50	2200	2400	2800	1800	2000	2200
51-55	2200	2400	2800	1600	1800	2200
56-60	2200	2400	2600	1600	1800	2200
61-65	2000	2400	2600	1600	1800	2000
66-70	2000	2200	2600	1600	1800	2000
71-75	2000	2200	2600	1600	1800	2000
76+	2000	2200	2400	1600	1800	2000

Table 2: Adapted from: Center for Nutrition Policy and Promotion, USDA

*Table based on healthy weight range

Sedentary- light physical activity involving day-to-day activities

Moderately active- equivalent of walking 1.5-3 miles per day along with day-to-day activities

Active- equivalent of walking more than 3 miles per day along with day-to-day activities

Here is the equation for those that love math. All of the calculations I learned in school were in kilograms and centimeters. Please don't ask me why, it's painful for me as well.

Conversions to kg and cm:

Weight: 1 kg = 2.2 lb   Weight in pounds_____ divided by 2.2 = _____ kg

Height: 2.54 cm = 1 in   Height in inches _____ times 2.54 =   _____ cm

Mifflin St. Jeor Equation [2]

Now that you have written down your weight in kg and height in cm, we can work on the equation.

Men: (10 x weight in kg) + (6.25 x height in cm) – (5 x age) + 5 = _____ kcal/day

Women: (10 x weight in kg) + (6.25 x height in cm) – (5 x age) – 161 = _____ kcal/day

Multiply your answer by the Activity Factor listed below.

*Ranges for sedentary based on ratio of total energy expenditure and basal energy expenditure.
*Ranges for other categories based on energy spent when walking at a particular pace.

Category	Values
Sedentary	1 – 1.39
Low activity	1.4 – 1.59
Active	1.6 – 1.89
Very active	1.9 – 2.5

_____ kcal/day x _____ activity factor = _____ kcal/day (calories needed each day)

For example: male, sedentary, 55 years old, 5'9", 205 pounds

1. 205 lb divided by 2.2 = 93.18 kg
2. 69 inches times 2.54 = 175.26 cm
3. (10 x 93.18 weight in kg) + (6.25 x 175.26 height in cm) − (5 x 55 age) + 5 = 1757.18 kcal/day
4. 1757.18 kcal x 1.3 sedentary range = 2284.33 = 2284 calories needed per day

The USDA food intake chart is helpful in comparing your intake to the recommendations. It also includes an extra equivalent chart just in case you want one. Take a look at your food and drink serving sizes that you filled out and compare it to this food intake chart.

Food Group Needs Per Day

Calorie Level	1,000	1,200	1,400	1,600	1,800	2,000	2,200	2,400	2,600	2,800	3,000	3,200
Grains (oz eq)	3 oz	4 oz	5 oz	5 oz	6 oz	6 oz	7 oz	8 oz	9 oz	10 oz	10 oz	10 oz
Vegetables (cups)	1 c	1 ½ c	1 ½ c	2 c	2 ½ c	2 ½ c	3 c	3 ½ c	3 ½ c	4 ½ c	4 c	4 c
Fruits (cups)	1 c	1 c	1 ½ c	1 ½ c	1 ½ c	2 c	2 c	2 c	2 c	2 ½ c	2 ½ c	2 ½ c
Protein (oz eq)	2 oz	3 oz	4 oz	5 oz	5 oz	5½oz	6 oz	6½oz	6½oz	7 oz	7 oz	7 oz
Dairy (cups)	2 c	2 ½ c	2 ½ c	3 c	3 c	3 c	3 c	3 c	3 c	3 c	3 c	3 c

Table 3: Adapted from: Center for Nutrition Policy and Promotion, USDA

oz eq = ounce equivalent

Now that I likely have you confused because, quite frankly, ounces and cups sometimes look like gibberish in comparison to how we think about food, here are some handy-dandy equivalent comparisons:

Grain group:

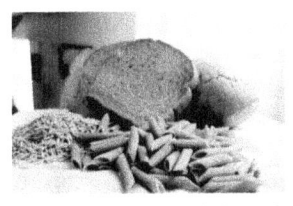

1 ounce equivalent =

1 slice of bread

1 cup of ready-to-eat cereal (one fist size)

½ cup of cooked rice, pasta, cereal (handful size)

**At least half of all grains consumed should be whole grains to help obtain adequate fiber intakes. (For example, brown rice, whole wheat bread, oatmeal, whole grain cereal, popcorn, whole wheat pasta.)

Vegetable group:

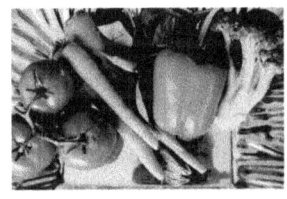

1 cup =

1 cup of raw or cooked vegetables (one fist size)

1 cup of vegetable juice

2 cups of raw leafy greens (2 fist size)

Table 4: Adapted from: Center for Nutrition Policy and Promotion, USDA

Fruit group:

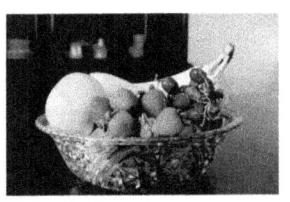

1 cup =

1 cup of fruit (one fist size)

1 cup of 100% fruit juice (fist size)

½ cup of dried fruit (handful)

Protein:

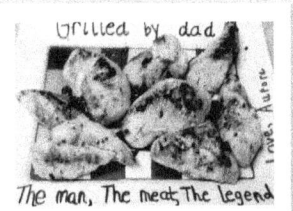

1 ounce equivalent =

1 ounce of lean meat, poultry, or seafood
   (3 oz is the size of the palm)

1 egg

1 Tb peanut butter (thumb size)

½ oz nuts or seeds (handful)

¼ cup beans (half of a handful)

Dairy:

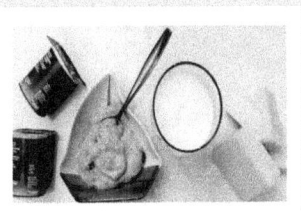

1 cup =

1 cup of milk or yogurt (fist size)

1 ½ oz of natural cheese (index finger size)

2 oz of processed cheese

Have you found anything that sticks out to you? Keep it in mind and, when we get to the nutrition counseling chapter, we'll pick it back up again.

To wrap up this chapter, let's talk about moderation. Who can forget the dreaded word "moderation?" That sounds like no fun at all. But let me tell you, I have been on this earth for a little while, and in order to create a sense of balance and well-being, moderation is the key. Here are some key points:

- Create a healthy balance of whole grains, vegetables, fruits, lean meats and dairy.
- Allow yourself some foods that may not be the healthiest for you. Just eat them in moderation with the healthier items being more predominant.
- Avoid the word "diet." Trust me. The moment you utter the word "diet" your brain goes into hyper drive and wants to eat everything in sight. Just stick with "I'm making better choices when I can."
- The moment you try and deprive yourself is the moment when that is all you can think of. So go ahead and allow yourself to avoid the stress and failure.
- Satiation. It's a great word and is all about listening to your body's cues. Stop eating the minute you feel full. Sometimes I have to tell myself, "This will NOT be the last time I eat this. There will be other chances on other days. I do NOT have to finish this all in one sitting."
- Allow yourself to succeed by choosing variety, balance and moderation!

As stated before, we'll talk more in-depth in the nutrition counseling session.

Chapter 2

Anthropometric Calculations

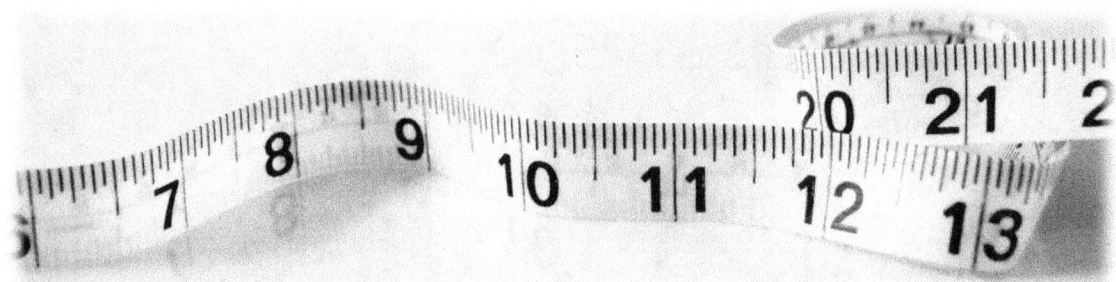

On the next few pages are a few chart calculations to do to see where you currently stand. These are not for shaming; it is simply for you to get an idea of where you are and where you would like to be.

Let's start with Body Mass Index (BMI).

This is a tool that helps measure body fat and can be used to determine whether you are at risk for future health problems such as Type 2 diabetes, high blood pressure and heart disease.

BMI ranges are not exact for those that are very muscular or for the elderly because increased or decreased muscle mass can distort the results. [3]

1. Go ahead and circle (or write down) your BMI category (normal, overweight, obese) below to see where you are and use it as motivation to get within a healthy range if you are not there already.

Body Mass Index (BMI) Chart

	Normal						Overweight					Obese					
BMI	**19**	**20**	**21**	**22**	**23**	**24**	**25**	**26**	**27**	**28**	**29**	**30**	**31**	**32**	**33**	**34**	**35**
Height (in)							**Weight (pounds)**										
58	91	96	100	105	110	115	119	124	129	134	138	143	148	153	158	162	167
59	94	99	104	109	114	119	124	128	133	138	143	148	153	158	163	168	173
60	97	102	107	112	118	123	128	133	138	143	148	153	158	163	168	174	179
61	100	106	111	116	122	127	132	137	143	148	153	158	164	169	174	180	185
62	104	109	115	120	126	131	136	142	147	153	158	164	169	175	180	186	191
63	107	113	118	124	130	135	141	146	152	158	163	169	175	180	186	191	197
64	110	116	122	128	134	140	145	151	157	163	169	174	180	186	192	197	204
65	114	120	126	132	138	144	150	156	162	168	174	180	186	192	198	204	210
66	118	124	130	136	142	148	155	161	167	173	179	186	192	198	204	210	216
67	121	127	134	140	146	153	159	166	172	178	185	191	198	204	211	217	223
68	125	131	138	144	151	158	164	171	177	184	190	197	203	210	216	223	230
69	128	135	142	149	155	162	169	176	182	189	196	203	209	216	223	230	236
70	132	139	146	153	160	167	174	181	188	195	202	209	216	222	229	236	243
71	136	143	150	157	165	172	179	186	193	200	208	215	222	229	236	243	250
72	140	147	154	162	169	177	184	191	199	206	213	221	228	235	242	250	258
73	144	151	159	166	174	182	189	197	204	212	219	227	235	242	250	257	265
74	148	155	163	171	179	186	194	202	210	218	225	233	241	249	256	264	272
75	152	160	168	176	184	192	200	208	216	224	232	240	248	256	264	272	279
76	156	164	172	180	189	197	205	213	221	230	238	246	254	263	271	279	287

Table 5: Adapted from: National Institutes of Health.

For a more comprehensive list, please visit:

https://www.nhlbi.nih.gov/health/educational/lose_wt/BMI/bmi_tbl.pdf

BMI Categories [3]	
Underweight	< 18.5
Normal weight	18.5 – 24.9
Overweight	25-29.9
Obesity	BMI of 30 or greater

Here is the calculation for those who love math.

BMI Equation [3]

$$BMI = \frac{(Weight\ in\ pounds)}{(Height\ in\ inches\ \times\ Height\ in\ inches)} \times 703 =$$

For example: male, sedentary, 55 years old, 5'9", 205 pounds:

$$\frac{(205\ lb)}{(69\ in\ \times\ 69\ in)} \times 703 = \frac{205}{4761} \times 703 = 30.27 = 30\ (obese)$$

Measuring your waist circumference is another way of determining if you are at risk for future health problems. So let's get out the measuring tape.

Waist Circumference [4]

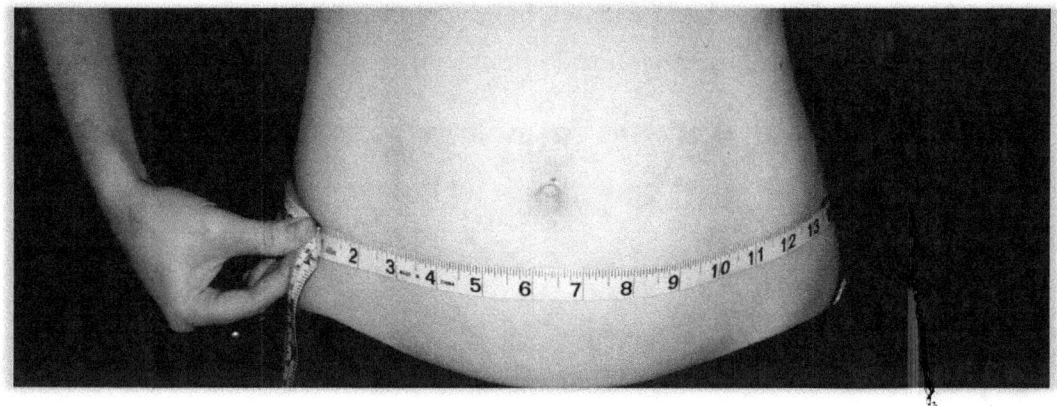

- Stand up and place a tape measure around your waist; just above the hipbone.
- Make sure the tape is horizontal around your waist.
- Make sure the tape is snug, but not pushing into the skin.
- Breathe out, then measure.

2. Write down your waist circumference : _____

A waist circumference of more than 40 inches for men may indicate future health problems.

A waist circumference of more than 35 inches for women may indicate future health problems. [4]

My goal for you in doing these calculations is to raise awareness.

You are welcome to skip over the body frame size/ideal weight calculations if you like. I do not obsess over numbers, and I do not expect you to either. But I did want to include them because some people just find it interesting and work better with numbers.

In order to determine your ideal weight, we need to figure out your body frame size. You will want to find your frame size because it may allow you an extra 10% in weight which will help your psyche and possibly your motivation.

Time to get out the trusty measuring tape again.

Body Frame Size

1. Measure your wrist where your watch band would normally go (at the smallest part, right above the styloid process on the ulna bone).

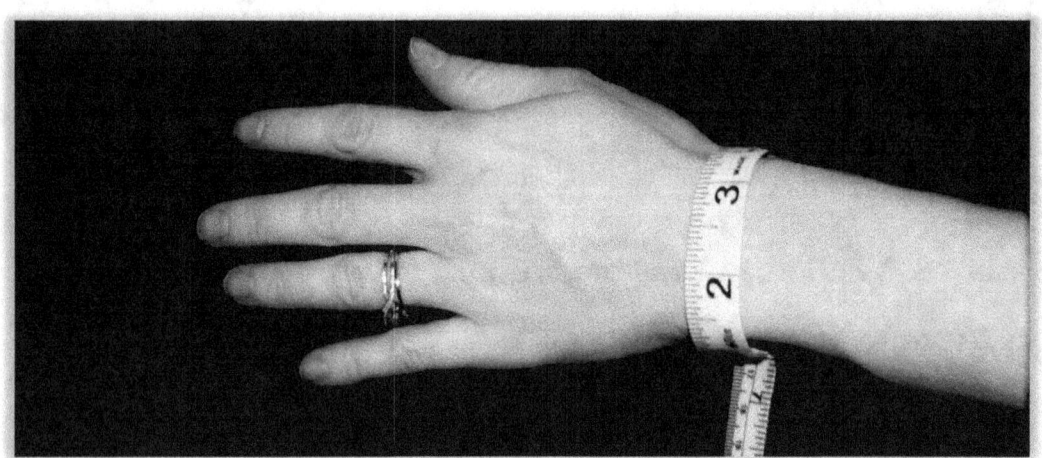

Women:		
Height under 5' 2"		
Frame Size	**Wrist Size (inches)**	
Small	Less than 5.5"	
Medium	5.5" - 5.75"	
Large	Over 5.75"	
Height 5'2" - 5'5"		
Frame Size	**Wrist Size**	
Small	Less than 6"	
Medium	6" - 6.25"	
Large	Over 6.25"	
Height over 5'5"		
Frame Size	**Wrist Size**	
Small	Less than 6.25"	
Medium	6.25" - 6.5"	
Large	Over 6.5"	

Men:	
Height over 5'5"	
Frame Size	**Wrist Size (inches)**
Small	5.5" - 6.5"
Medium	6.5" - 7.5"
Large	Over 7.5"

2. Circle or write down your body frame size depending on your sex. We're going to use it in a minute.

Let's move on to ideal weight. The Hamwi equation is not perfect. None of them are, but it is used often and can be a good guide.

3. Calculate your ideal weight using the calculation below.

Hamwi Calculation for Ideal Weight [5]

Men:
<ul><li>106 lbs for first 5 feet of height and 6 lb per inch over 5 feet.</li><li>Add or subtract 10% depending on frame size (for a small frame size, you may want to subtract 10% and for a large frame size you may want to add 10%.)</li></ul>
Women:
<ul><li>100 lbs for first 5 feet of height and 5 lbs per inch over 5 feet.</li><li>Add or subtract 10% depending on frame size (for a small frame size, you may want to subtract 10% and for a large frame size you may want to add 10%.)</li></ul>

For example:

Male, 205 pounds, 5'9", large frame size.

Short version:

106 + (9 x 6) = 160 lb

*NOTE: a 10% plus or minus is allowed depending on frame size

160 x .10 = 16

160 + 16 = 176 lb ideal weight

Long version:

106 for first 5 feet =   106

9 inches over 5 feet x 6 from calculation =   9 x 6 = 54

106 + 54 = 160 lb

*NOTE: a 10% plus or minus is allowed depending on frame size.

160 x .10 = 16

160 + 16 = 176 lb ideal weight.

---

205 lb current weight − 176 lb ideal weight = 29

This client is 29 pounds over his ideal weight.

Okay, okay, enough with the calculations!!

Let's move on to chapter 3 and try to understand some factors that might be influencing your weight.

Chapter 3

Factors Influencing Weight

Maybe, just maybe, there is something or someone out there to blame other than yourself for any extra weight you might be struggling with. Well, you're in luck, possibly. Or maybe you just eat too much and the idea of exercise makes you want to scream. Either way, let's talk about this!

1. Diet

A diet high in fast food, high-fat foods and large portion sizes can lead to eventual weight problems. [6] I'm not saying that you have to cut out these foods; that would be torture and unrealistic for most of us. I'm saying that we need to become comfortable with the words "moderation" and "balance". Try to think of ways that you can make better choices when you are at a fast food restaurant.

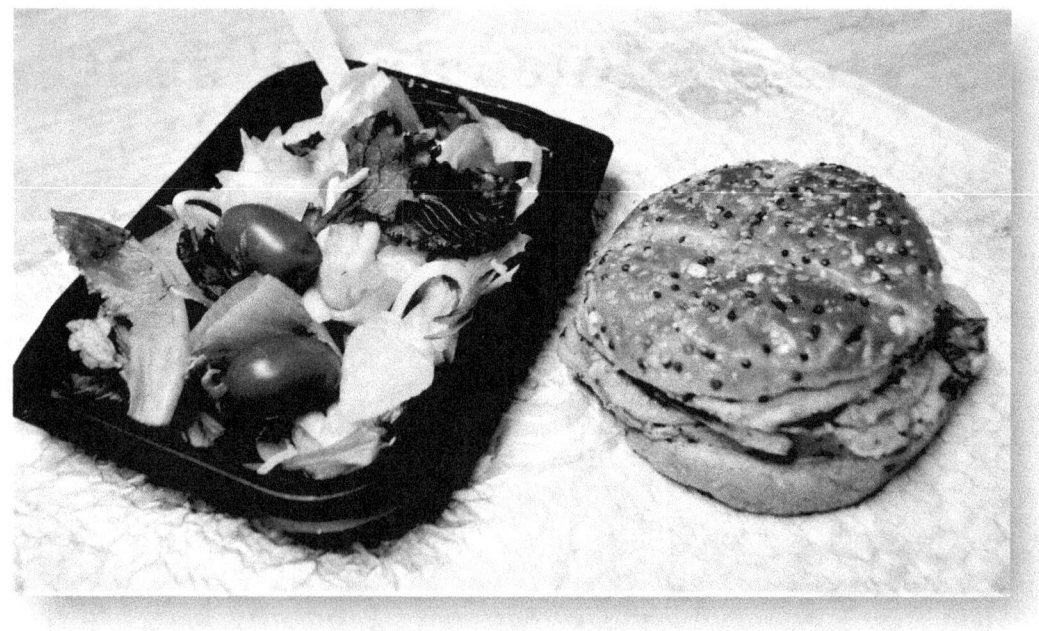

What ways can you help lower your portion sizes when at restaurants or at home? You don't have to try and implement this right away, we'll use this information later. List them out here:

_____

_____

_____

_____

Some examples might include:

> • Choose grilled items.
> • Order a small fry with a side salad instead of a large fry.
> • Use low fat dressing.
> • Fill your plate with more vegetables or salad rather than extra pizza slices.
> • Swap the milkshake for a fruit parfait, small ice cream cone or small frozen yogurt.
> • Ask for a to-go bag with your meal and immediately put half of your restaurant dinner in the to-go bag.
> • Share a meal or dessert.
> • Order refreshing ice water or unsweetened iced tea in place of soda.

The possibilities are endless and you can still enjoy your favorite foods while just cutting back on how much you eat. Really and truly understand that if you eat more food than you can burn off, then your weight is going to eventually increase over time.

2. Activity Level

When asked, most people draw a hard line about their love or hatred of exercise. And that's okay. When you are initially losing weight, what and how much you eat is the main contributor to your success at weight loss. [7] Exercise becomes most important once you have lost the weight and are in the maintenance phase.

Keep in mind, though, that people who are consistently sedentary tend to weigh more.

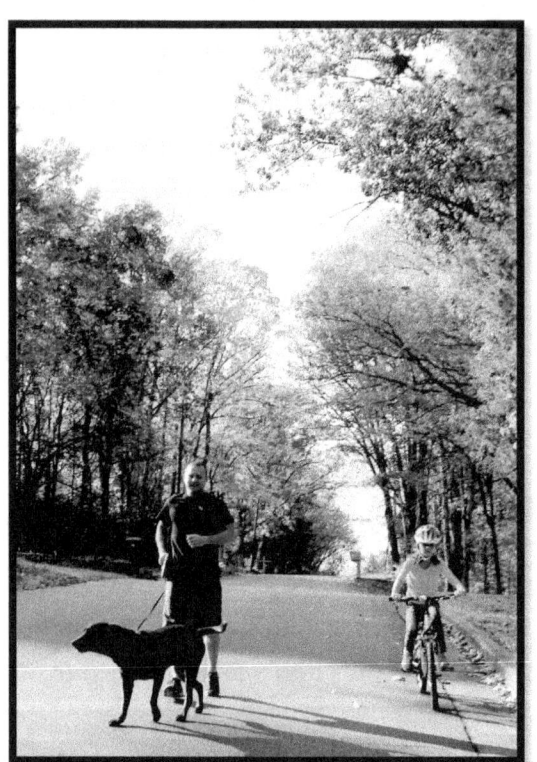

And there's good news for those that hate exercise! According to the American Heart Association (AHA), a brisk walk is just as good as running.[8] So, for those of you who think you have to go extreme-o in order to get health benefits (and the whole idea just turns you off), you don't! Just get up and get moving after dinner or lunch a few times a week! [8]

What are some activities that you enjoy that can get you active and be a good role model for your family? List them below:

_____

_____

_____

_____

Activities such as raking leaves, gardening, and cleaning the house can be included. They can also be therapeutic and meditative, while allowing for increased activity.

Some companies even give incentives to employees for how many calories they burn. Some people choose to just take a stroll in their work clothes during their lunch break.

If moderation is your trouble, like it is for my husband, and you tend to go back for seconds at dinner, then exercise might be key for you (and also filling up on vegetables). My husband would rather exercise more in order to be able to eat more, and it works for him.

When he can't exercise, he tries to fill up his plate with more vegetables to help him feel more full and lower the chances of going back in the kitchen for seconds.

3. Genetics

The storage of fat in your body is greatly influenced by genetics. This includes how much fat you store and where it is stored. [9]

While your chances of being overweight are higher if one more both of your parents are overweight, that does not mean that you will automatically be overweight because environment also plays a large part in the family link and that part is more controllable.

4. Environment

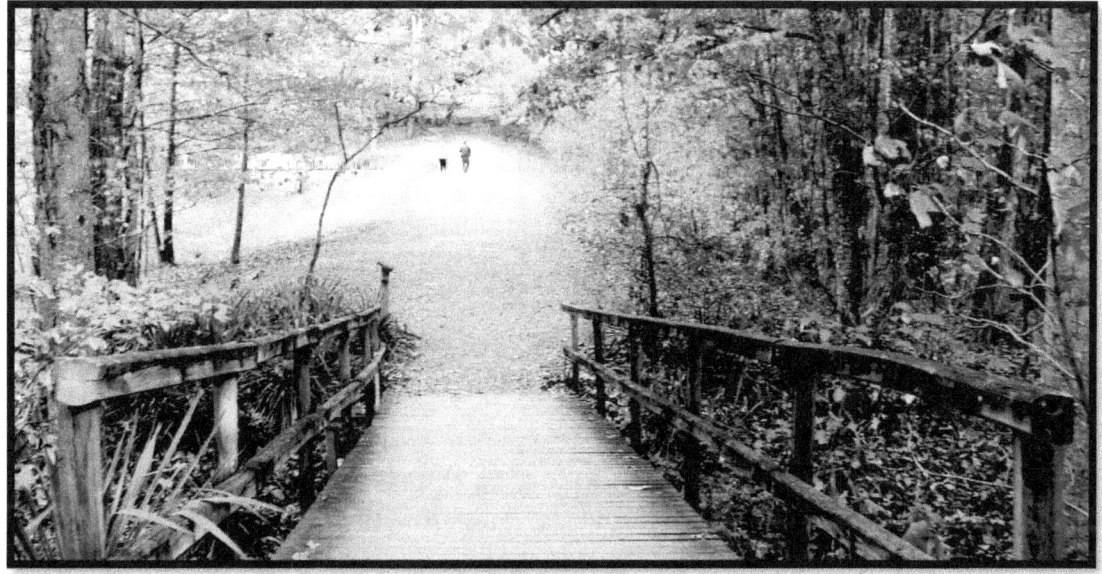

Eating and exercise habits are formed early in life and are greatly influenced by family. This may have had a positive influence for some and that is great! If not, that is okay. It is not too late to form new and healthier habits. As an adult you can take control of your life.

You can also ask those around you to be supportive and understanding (and even join you!) as you go through the journey to better health.

What are some positive eating or physical activity habits that you already have or that you can create for yourself or with your family?

_____

_____

_____

_____

5. Psychological Roadblocks

Ah, stress and anxiety. Sometimes it gets to us. Sometimes we overeat to try and cope.

Here are some great tips to help overcome stress:

Reducing Stress
1. Learn to say "no."
2. Organize. Checking off tasks as they are completed helps with a sense of control and a reduction of anxiety.
3. Exercise. Activities such as walking and swimming help relieve tension.
4. Have a positive attitude. Surround yourself with positive people.
5. Relaxation and meditation.
6. Sleep. Getting enough sleep helps put thoughts into a better perspective.
7. Healthy eating for the body.
8. Stop being so hard on yourself. Dust off your boots and move on.
9. Strive at being a good friend and surrounding yourself with good friends.
10. Accept yourself; talents and limitations included.
11. Laugh!
12. Take deep breaths.
13. Forgive. Holding on to anger and grudges hurts you way more than it hurts them.

Table 7: Adapted from: Bauer Nutrition Skill Development

Let's take a minute to bring awareness to emotional eating.

Bringing awareness to your life

1.   Think about yesterday and what you had to eat and drink. Write it down:
2.   What were you feeling at the time of eating each food? Write the feeling next to the item. Maybe you were bored, stressed, angry or lonely. Write it down. What about today?

_____   _____   _____

_____   _____   _____

_____   _____   _____

_____   _____   _____

_____   _____   _____

_____   _____   _____

_____   _____   _____

_____   _____   _____

_____   _____   _____

_____   _____   _____

Are you noticing any patterns?

Keeping a food diary can help you identify patterns in your behavior and mood and how it affects your food choices.

Alternative Behaviors

If you wrote down a negative emotion next to a food item, what is a positive alternative solution instead of eating? WebMD has some great suggestions. I'll list them. [10]

"Frustrated because you feel like you're not in control? Go for a walk on a path you choose."

"Hurt by a co-worker's mean comments? Take it out on a punching bag or make a plan for how you're going to talk it out."

"Bored? Distract yourself by calling a friend or surfing the Internet."

    3.   What are some other positive behaviors that you can choose instead of eating?

_____

_____

_____

_____

Exercise!

If you need more reasons to stop hating exercise, then you're in luck. Exercise decreases anxiety, decreases stress and it can improve your mood. [11] Studies show that even 5 minutes of exercise can decrease anxiety! [11] It can also help improve self-esteem and sleep. We'll talk more about exercise in Chapter 17!

6. Medications

Certain medications may lead to weight gain. Some of these include medications for diabetes, depression, seizures, allergies, steroid therapy or hormone therapy. Do not stop taking a medication before consulting with your doctor. However, if you have noticed a change in your weight after taking any medications, then talk to your doctor and they may be able to recommend an alternative for you that is either "weight-neutral" or can promote weight loss. [12]

7. Medical Conditions

When the thyroid gland doesn't produce enough thyroid hormone, hypothyroidism may result.[13] The American Thyroid Association (ATA) states that hypothyroidism is a condition that affects approximately 12% of Americans and 5 times more cases are seen in women than in men. [14] Hypothyroidism can cause weight gain as well as feelings of being tired and weak.

Cushing's syndrome may develop if the adrenal glands produce too much cortisol and can cause weight gain. [13]

5-10% of women of childbearing age may develop polycystic ovarian syndrome and obesity is common with this syndrome. [13]

8. Sleep

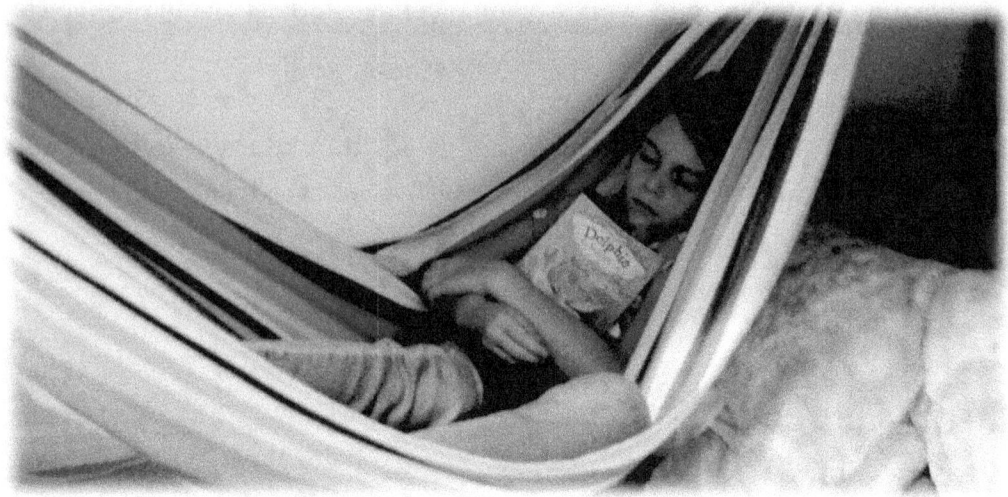

Sleeeep. One of my favorite words and activities and is so very important for you. If you are not getting enough sleep, then that may eventually contribute to weight gain. We'll talk in detail about hormones in a later chapter, but it is important to point out that sleep plays an important role in the hormonal balance of appetite and hunger. [15] As reported by the National Institutes of Health (NIH), those who are not getting enough rest tend to be more prone to obesity due to the body's desire to eat more calories and carbohydrates. [15]

9. Set-Point Theory

This is a very interesting theory by Bennit and Gurin, and I have seen it play out multiple times. It simply means that our bodies want to maintain a certain set point for fat. [16]

When we attempt to severely lower our calories long-term, the body thinks it is being starved and will actually lower your metabolism. At a certain point, this makes it very hard to lose more weight and some may experience a "plateau period."

If you are exercising, then mixing up your exercise routine may help lower the set point and overcome the plateau, so that is good news. If you aren't exercising, now might be a good time to start, no matter how slow.

A severe restriction of calories is never the long-term answer and some may even gain weight because certain hormones kick in that cause us to feel hungry all the time.

If you can't tell, I discourage traditional dieting.

According to the most reputable sources for health and wellness, such as the U.S. Department of Agriculture (USDA), Mayo Clinic, and American Heart Association (AHA), the most promising way to lose weight AND ACTUALLY KEEP IT OFF is to create small, realistic goals and follow through with them. [17, 18, 19] Although a slow process, conquering these goals one at a time and over an extended amount of time helps build better eating habits, a healthy balance for a lifetime and inevitable weight loss.

So stay tuned. We will be discussing those details in the nutrition counseling portion in the next chapter.

Chapter 4

Health and Weight Management Counseling

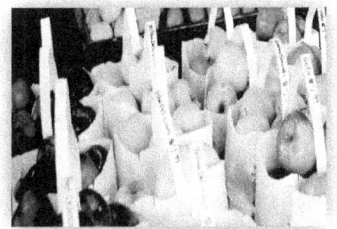 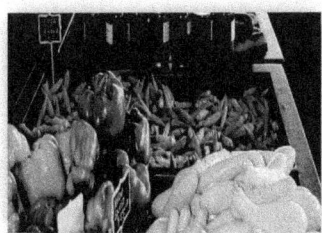 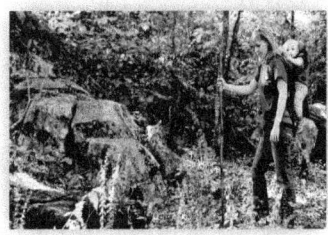

Remember Chapter 1 where you wrote down your foods/drinks over the last 24 hours and we talked about areas that stuck out to you that you might want to work on? Go back and take a look at that list, please.

If you didn't do it, then that's okay, just go back to chapter 1 and work through that chapter and come back here when you're done.

Let's make another list. Can you tell I'm a big list-maker? Lists do wonders for organization, so I highly recommend them.

1. Using your food and drink intake information from Chapter 1, list out any food groups that you can work on. For example, if you are supposed to get 3 cups of milk per day and you get 1, add that to the list. If you know that your fats, sweets and dessert intakes are excessive, write that down.
2. Now think of your overall lifestyle habits. Do you eat at fast food and/or sit-down restaurants multiple nights a week? Do you smoke? Drink more than 1 alcoholic drink per day for women and 2 drinks per day for men? If you answered yes to any of those, write it down. Do you exercise? If you answered no, write it down.

Basically, write down any unhealthy habits that may be contributing to your weight problem:

——————————— ——————————— ———————————

——————————— ——————————— ———————————

——————————— ——————————— ———————————

——————————— ——————————— ———————————

DO NOT WORRY, you are not alone in your potentially long list of bad habits. We are NOT going to tackle all of them at once. This just helps us organize our problems so that we can tackle them one by one.

3. You know what, let's also list all of the positive health habits we have. Do you drink plenty of water? Write that down. Do you love whole grains and try to eat them as often as possible? Do you make time for a brisk walk? Write all of your healthy habits down:

_____	_____	_____
_____	_____	_____
_____	_____	_____
_____	_____	_____
_____	_____	_____

Take a minute to congratulate yourself on the positive aspects of your diet and lifestyle. If you already have some positive food habits, then you know that you can create more for yourself. You will find that, over time, your list of bad behaviors will slowly be conquered and you will add the positive equivalent to your positive health habit list.

Okay, back to the tough part. Let's take a close look at our bad habits list.

4. Pick only one or two items from the bad habits list that you think are most realistic to actually change and list them:

- _____

- _____

Never underestimate the ruler. Use this "**Readiness to Change**" assessment ruler, from Prochaska and DiClemente, and write down your readiness to change number next to the bad habit.

1	2	3	4	5	6	7	8	9	10	11	12

1= not ready
12= ready and motivated

If your number fell between 1-4, then you are considered "not motivated and not ready." [20]

If your number fell between 5-8, then you are "unsure, low confidence."

If your number is 9-12, then you are "motivated, confident and ready."

Since you are taking the time to read this book, I believe it is safe to say that you can find at least one, if not more, habits that you are motivated and ready to change. So go ahead and skip over to the 9-12 (motivated, confident and ready) area.

However, over the months, as you progress through your nutrition goals, you may find you are stuck in trying to find motivation with one or two goals. If that time comes, take a look at 1-4 (not motivated and not ready) and 5-8 (unsure, low confidence) in order to provide some tips to help in overcoming your barriers and motivating yourself to change.

1-4- Not Motivated, Not Ready

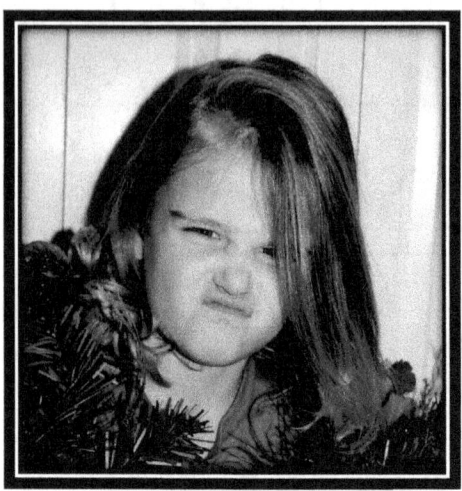

Take a look at your bad habit. Think about some consequences if you don't change your bad habit. Think about some benefits if you do make the change.

Let's say you are eating fast food multiple nights a week and you want to cut it down to only once or twice a week. One consequence of not changing includes a high salt intake, which can lead to high blood pressure. A high fat intake through high fat meats and fried foods can lead to heart disease. The high calorie content can lead to excessive weight gain. Some benefits of making certain fast food changes include lowering blood pressure, lowering risk of heart disease and losing weight or avoiding extra weight gain. It may also include knowing that you are making healthier choices for the entire family, which can impact them positively for the rest of their lives.

 If you are still not ready, then just know that you need to be thinking about this and at some point you will need to change if it starts to affect your health.

5-8 Unsure, Low Confidence

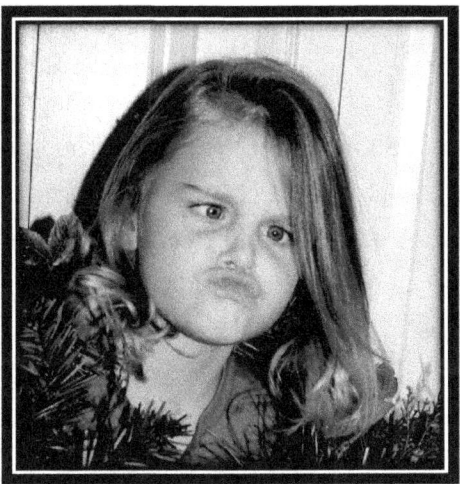

Think about why you are unsure about making the change. Are there a lot of barriers that you would have to overcome and it makes you feel overwhelmed? Let's talk about some of those barriers. What are the barriers to you achieving your goal? List them here:

_____ _____

_____ _____

_____ _____

What are some ways that you can overcome those barriers? List them out:

_____ _____

_____ _____

_____ _____

Let's use the fast food example again. Say some barriers include that you are toting kids around all evening to sports and don't have time to cook a meal at home. That is a legitimate barrier.

Now how do we overcome that barrier? If you aren't able to cook ahead of time, then maybe making healthier choices at the fast food restaurant is an option. What are some healthy options at each fast food restaurant you frequent? Or maybe sometimes you can go to a fast food restaurant that offers healthier options, like Subway®?

The point is that YOU need to decide that you need to change and YOU need to be the one that comes up with solutions that will work for you. I can't make you change, and I can't tell you what to change or how to make those changes. You are in control of your future, so take the reins! And before you know it, you will have a list of ways to combat any barriers you may come across and will be well on your way to success!

9-12 Motivated, Confident, Ready

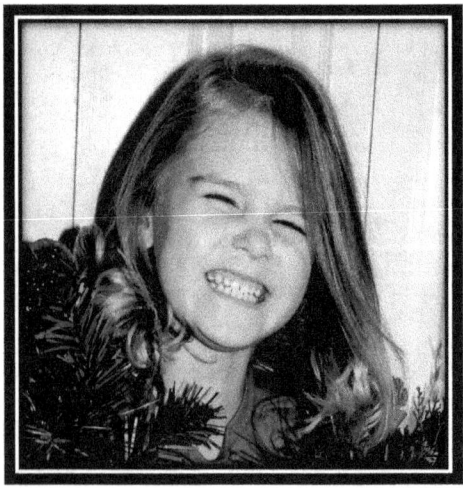

Good for you for being ready to making positive changes!

Remember that list where we talked about all the positive health habits you have? Review those again, and congratulate yourself again. Change does not occur overnight, but give yourself some credit for what you already do and just know that you have the ability and motivation to add to your list of positive health habits.

Now let's get down to business: goal writing.

As clinical psychologist Fitzhugh Dodson said, "Goals that are not written down are just wishes." [21]

1. Take one of your bad habits and write it down:

_____

For example: "I need 2 fruits per day, but I only get about 2 fruits per week."

2. Now write down a general and broad goal that will change that negative into a positive.

_____

For example: "I will eat more fruit in place of chips."

That is a great goal, let's just fine tune it.

Use the SMART objectives, developed by the Centers for Disease Control (CDC) Division for Heart Disease and Stroke Prevention (DHDSP), when goal setting. [22]

SMART Objectives for Goal Setting

- Specific
- Measurable
- Action-oriented
- Realistic
- Time frame

---

3. Be EXTREMELY specific. Write down EXACTLY how you are going to achieve this goal. Make it short, specific, achievable and include a time frame!

_____

The actual goal might go something like this: "I will eat 1 fruit for my 10 am snack each day for 2 weeks."

After a while you will start doing that goal without even thinking about it and you will be replacing unhealthy habits for healthier habits!

4. Next: Write down your final goal on a piece of paper. Put it front and center at your desk or by the fruit bowl or tape it to your front door. Add 14 little squares (or for how many ever days your goal is for) and each day, check it off.

These goals may seem minute, but I am telling you, slowly replacing unhealthy habits for healthy ones will pay off in the long run. These health goals will lead to eventual (and long lasting) weight loss when you combine multiple positive health habits over time. AND you will decrease your risk of nutrition-related diseases AND you will feel better about yourself. Win all around!

Evaluate

Once you have conquered that goal, step it up once more. Keep eating your 1 piece of fruit at snack time. While maintaining your original goal, make a new goal that states something like, "I will drink 8 oz of 100% juice with my breakfast each morning for 2 weeks."

Juice is not the best source of fruit because it typically lacks fiber. But just remember that you have to start somewhere. In the future, if you decide adding fiber to your diet is a goal, then you can replace the orange juice with an orange or buy full pulp orange juice. Anyway, I think you get the gist!

A Few Tips for Your Journey

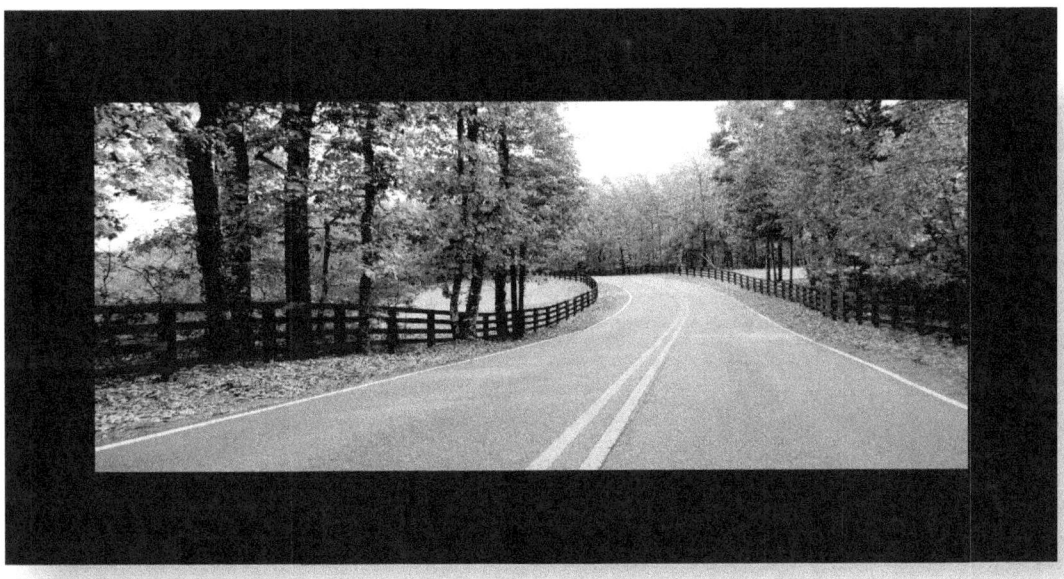

Do yourself a favor and take your time.

If you mess up on your goal, don't beat yourself up. This is not about perfection. Get right back on track! Those who strive for perfection, try to do too much at once or are too restrictive are usually the ones that eventually gain the weight back or give up all together.

This is about taking it slow. If you mess up, take a look at what was going on at the time that it happened. Assess the situation, look at ways to prevent it in the future, and then get right back on track!

Then keep on with it. And keep reading. You have more chapters to go and just keeping in the healthful eating mind frame will help keep you motivated!

Chapter 5

Nutrition-Related Diseases and Normal Lab Ranges

"Let food be thy medicine and medicine be thy food."
-Hippocrates

Now that we have made a goal for ourselves and written it down, let's spend this chapter talking about WHY it is so important to maintain a healthy weight and how foods interact with our bodies for long-term health. These reasons will be discussed in the following chapters. I hope you read through them to gain a better understanding of how food interacts in our bodies and why nutrition is the main point, rather than just cutting back on calories.

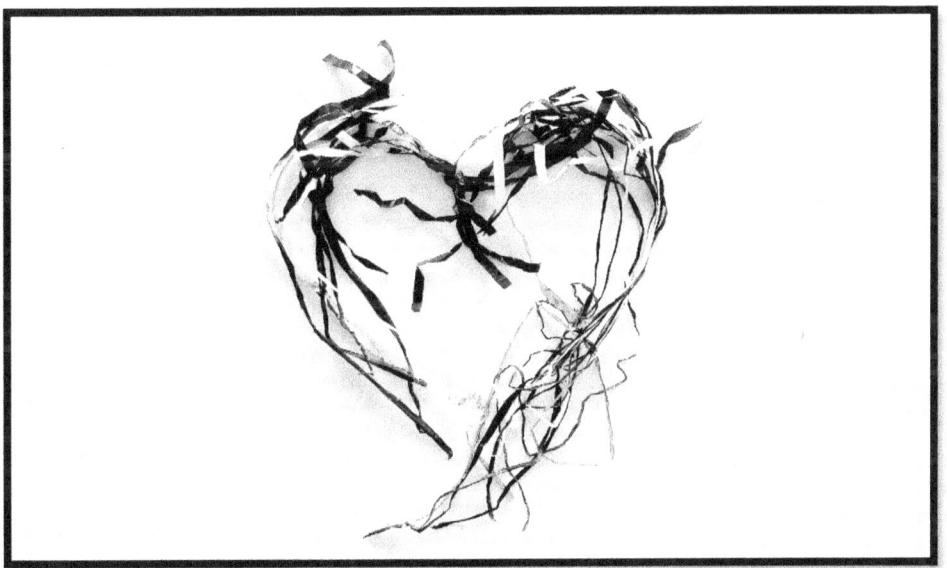

Let's start with some statistics to put things into perspective:

- The Centers for Disease Control (CDC) reports that overweight and obesity contributes to 4 of the 6 leading causes of death. [23]

These deaths are considered chronic diseases and include heart disease, cancer, stroke and diabetes. And guess what? They are the MOST PREVENTABLE!!! [23]

Side note: <u>Metabolic syndrome</u> is when you have a cluster of 3 or more risk factors, such as large waistline, high triglyceride level, low levels of HDL (high-density lipoprotein) level, high blood pressure or high fasting blood sugar. [24] These greatly increase your risk of heart disease or other health problems.

Below is a list of the number of Americans diagnosed with chronic disease due to diet and inactivity: [25]

1. Overweight/obese : 142,000,000. That's approximately 66% of the population!
2. High blood pressure: 73,000,000
3. Diabetes: 24,000,000.
4. Coronary heart disease: 16,000,000
5. Cancer: 11,000,000
6. Stroke: 5,800,000.

- I stated it above, but it bears repeating: Overweight and obese adults make up approximately 66% of the American population. [25]
- 1 in 3 children and young adults are obese and 1 in 5 are overweight. [25]
- Approximately 30% of cancers are nutrition- and activity-related. [26]

Nutrition Statistics:

Only 10% of Americans adhere to healthy eating, according to the National Alliance for Nutrition and Activity (NANA). [25] Diets high in saturated fat, trans fat, salt and refined sugars contribute to health problems while diets high in fruits, vegetables and whole grains contribute to DECREASING chronic-related health problems.

Exercise Statistics:

NANA also states that only half of Americans get the recommended amount of exercise each week. [25] Regular physical activity helps prevent chronic health problems such as heart disease, certain cancers, diabetes, high blood pressure and obesity.

Alright, now that I have thrown some scary numbers around, let's talk about prevention. I cannot and will not diagnose or treat diseases, but I can and LOVE to discuss prevention!

Note: This discussion will be pretty broad, but will be covered in detail in later chapters when we discuss macronutrients, micronutrients, functional foods and exercise.

Heart Disease

With 16 million diagnoses and 652,091 deaths in 2010, heart disease is the No. 1 killer in America. [25]

We can reduce our chances of getting heart disease through fruits, vegetables, whole grains, omega-3 fats and lean meats.

We will talk more about this in detail in later chapters of macronutrients.

An increase in exercise and a decrease in cholesterol, stress and tobacco also contribute to lowered rates of heart disease.

Some typical tests to look for and keep within a normal range:

Tests	Information	Normal Range
Blood pressure	Important indicator of heart disease	120/80
Total cholesterol	Important indicator of heart disease	<200 mg/dL
Low density lipoprotein (LDL)	High amount can cause fatty deposits in arteries (atherosclerosis)	<130 mg/dL
High density lipoprotein (HDL)	Helps lower unhealthy LDL levels	>60 mg/dL
Triglycerides	High amount typically means you are consuming more calories than you are burning	<150 mg/dL
C-reactive protein	Indicator of inflammation, which can lead to atherosclerosis	<1 mg/dL

Table 8: Adapted from: Mayo Clinic

Cancer

As mentioned before, approximately 30% of cancers are nutrition-related. [26]

Plant-based foods, such as fruits, vegetables and whole grains can lower the risk of stomach and colon cancer.

While the studies are mixed, a lowered fat intake may help lower the risk of prostate, colon, rectum and uterine cancers.

Limiting alcohol may lower the risk of oral and esophageal cancer. [27]

Maintaining a healthy weight may help lower the risk for prostate, colon, rectum, uterine, ovarian, breast, esophageal and gallbladder cancers. [27]

Stroke

Stroke can be caused by factors such as high blood pressure and atherosclerosis (a fatty plaque buildup in the arteries) .[28]

A regular intake of fruits, vegetables and whole grains can help reduce the risk of stroke.

Limiting salt, solid fats, added sugars, calories, tobacco and alcohol can also reduce your risk.

Increasing physical activity is also known to lower stroke risk. [28]

Diabetes

There are two types of diabetes. [29]

Type 1 diabetes is genetic and occurs when the pancreas produces too little insulin in order to regulate blood sugar levels appropriately.

Type 2 diabetes occurs when cell receptors are overused so insulin is not utilized properly.

Since the rate of diagnosis in children is now 46%, affecting adults and children almost equally, it is no longer called "adult onset" diabetes. [25]

This is sad information, but there is hope! The most important factor in preventing Type 2 diabetes is weight control through a healthy diet and exercise. [30] And we are in control of that!

Harvard University reports that losing 7-10% of your current weight can cut your Type 2 diabetes chances in half. [30]

Whole grains help protect against diabetes while sugary drinks, unhealthy fats, red meat and processed meat increase the risk of diabetes.

We will talk about sources of fats and meats when we cover macronutrients.

Some typical tests to look for and keep within a normal range:

Tests	Information	Normal Range
Glycated hemoglobin (A1C) test	Measures average blood sugar levels from the past 2-3 months	<5.7 %
Random blood sugar test	Randomly tested to determine sugar values	<125 md/dL
Fasting blood sugar test	Taken after an overnight fast	<100 mg/dL
Oral glucose tolerance test	Taken after an overnight fast and after drinking a sugary liquid	<140 mg/dL

Table 9: Adapted from: Mayo Clinic

Overweight and Obesity

Shall I repeat what we discussed? You bet. Overweight and obesity can lead to Type 2 diabetes, heart disease, high blood pressure, certain cancers and stroke. Basically: death.

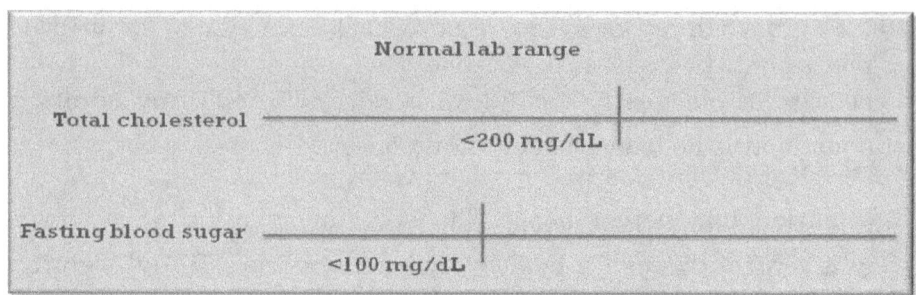

Is it preventable? Typically, yes, through healthy eating and exercise.

We talked about setting our goals earlier in chapter 4. As you begin replacing unhealthy choices with more healthy ones, you will find that your empty calories, overall calories, fat and salt intake will decrease.

This can help naturally lower your weight.   Naturally.   Gradually.   Steadily.

These are key words because those who take their time with their health and weight loss goals are much more successful in KEEPING IT OFF!! [31]

And just think, only a 5-10% weight reduction can reduce your risk of obesity-related chronic diseases and help improve your blood pressure, blood cholesterol and blood sugar results. [31]

We're not counting calories or weight here, but as time goes on, you will find that your goals will naturally help you lose weight.

Teressa Wray, RDN, LDN, my kind and patient preceptor from my internship days, had a client that was able to lose weight simply by following through with the goal of lowering his soda intake. For example, say you drink 2 sodas per day, which is 300 calories total. Let's also say your chosen goal is to replace 1 soda for 1 glass of ice water or unsweetened iced tea. That is a 150 calorie savings per day. Then let's say you conquer that goal in a few weeks and add on to it. So now you want to replace the 2nd soda with unsweet tea. That is another 150 calorie savings per day. So, over a matter of a month, you can potentially save yourself 300 calories per day. Easy-peasy.

Since 3,500 calories equals 1 pound, [31] you will be able to lose 1 pound approximately every 11 days just by switching out 2 sodas with healthier options! That may not sound like a lot, but I'm telling you, SLOW AND STEADY WINS THE RACE!!

Again, please do not think I want you to start counting calories. It's quite the opposite, actually. The focus is on healthy habits and a healthy lifestyle. You won't need to count calories to start seeing a positive difference in your life emotionally and physically.

Speaking of healthier habits, I am so grateful that there is an exercise area in the same church building as my daughter's karate. It allows me to slowly walk my pregnant butt on the treadmill while she is at karate class.

So I have started a new goal for myself: "I will walk for 30 minutes on the treadmill on Tuesdays and Thursdays for 3 weeks."

Once I get that goal down pat, I will either just be satisfied with that goal and keep it up or add a new goal such as walking for 30 minutes while she is in ballet or use that time to use the weight machines. I'll figure that out when it comes time. Right now I have my goal and will be working on it just as you are working on yours! I have figured out how to use my surroundings and circumstances to work my goal into my life and overcome any barriers. And that's how it works. A simple, achievable goal that you can slowly build upon to help achieve your overall health and weight loss goals. Anyway, I digressed.

Some typical tests to look for and keep within a normal range:

Tests	Information	Normal Range
Body Mass Index (BMI)	Measure of body fat based on height and weight	18.5-24.9
Waist circumference (WC)	Screens for health risks related to overweight and obesity	Women: <35 inches Men: <40 inches
Total cholesterol	Important indicator of heart disease	<200 mg/dL
Fasting blood sugar test	Taken after an overnight fast	<100 mg/dL
Thyroid test	Measures thyroid stimulating hormone (TSH) in blood	0.4-4 mIU/L

Table 10: Adapted from: Mayo Clinic

Let's move on shall we? Macronutrients are up next: protein, carbohydrates and fats; how they work in our body, what are some good sources and how much we need.

Chapter 6

Macronutrients: Protein

Protein

I won't go into detail with chemistry, nutritional biochemistry and elementary organic chemistry. However, since I did have to take them, I will cover the macronutrients section in a broad, thus less painful, way throughout these next few chapters.

Some of this will be a review for you and some of it will likely be new information. Let's start with protein.

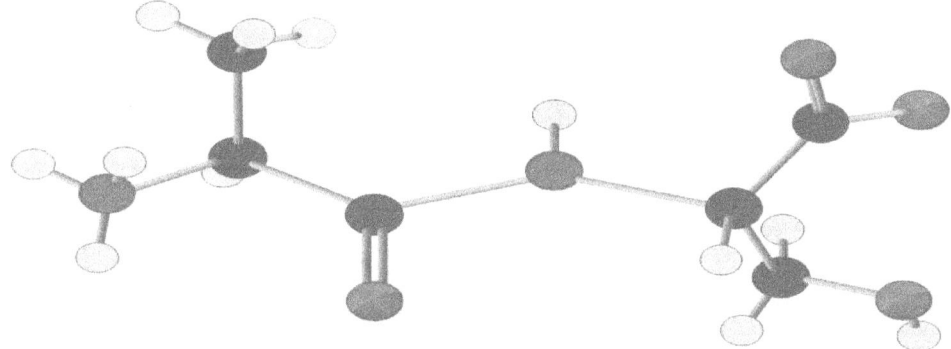

Peptide bond of amino acids alanine and serine

Amino acids are the building blocks of protein.

There are 20 amino acids and the body cannot make 9 of them, so those 9 have to be eaten in foods. [32]

Those that the body can make on its own are called <u>nonessential amino acids</u>.

The 9 amino acids that MUST be eaten through foods are called <u>essential amino acids</u>. They include valine, methionine, histidine, lysine, phenylalanine, leucine, isoleucine, tryptophan and arginine. A cute mnemonic, from *Metabolism and Nutrition*, to help remember them (if you care) is Very Many Hairy Little Pigs Live In Torrid Argentine. [33]

Each amino acid has a different chemical property and they link together through peptide bonds to form a protein molecule. [32]

Why is protein so important, you ask? Here's why:

Protein is required for the <u>structure and function</u> of the body and is found in muscle, bone, skin and hair. [34]

<u>Chemical reactions</u>, such as food breakdown and blood clotting, are constantly taking place in your body and are fueled by protein enzymes.[34]

Protein and Weight Management

While that is interesting from a health standpoint, those that are on a weight loss journey might find this information, from *Organic and Biochemistry for Today*, a little more interesting: [35]

Protein has the <u>BEST ability to beat hunger</u>. Since protein is such a complex molecule, it takes much longer to break down in the body (thermic effect), which provides a longer-lasting source of energy.

Protein can slightly <u>boost the metabolism</u>. By eating more protein, you are burning more calories due to the thermic effect discussed above.

Protein triggers a <u>hormone appetite-suppressant</u>. We will talk about these hormones in a later chapter, so stay tuned.

Protein can help <u>maintain lean body mass</u> when losing weight.

 *The following tables of portion sizes and grams are purely informational. I am not asking you to keep track of every bite of food you take and every gram it consists of.

Common Sources of Protein

Animal sources provide all of the essential amino acids and include meat, fish, poultry, eggs and dairy. They are a <u>complete protein</u> or <u>high biological value proteins</u>. [36]

Sources of High Biological Value Proteins

Animal Product	Portion Size	Grams of Protein
Beef, lean	3 oz (size of your palm)	26 grams
Tuna, in water	3 oz	22 grams
Hamburger, lean	3 oz	24 grams
Chicken, no skin	3 oz	28 grams
Lamb	3 oz	23 grams
Pork chop, lean	3 oz	22 grams
Salmon, broiled	3 oz	22 grams
Shrimp, broiled	3 oz	20 grams
Lobster, steamed	3 oz	16 grams
Egg	1 medium	6 grams
(*1 egg per day will not increase the risk of heart disease.) [37]		
Greek yogurt, nonfat	6 oz	18 grams
Cottage cheese	4 oz	14 grams
Regular yogurt, nonfat	1/2 cup	5 grams
Milk, skim	1 cup (size of fist)	8 grams
String cheese, skim	1 oz (size of thumb)	6 grams

Table 11: Adapted from: Today's Dietitian

While these vegetarian products are not considered as high quality as animal proteins, they are still complete proteins:

Plant Product	Portion Size	Grams of Protein
Soy, tofu	3 oz.	8 grams
Quinoa	½ cup (handful size)	4 grams

Table 12: Adapted from: Soy Foods Assn and the Vegetarian Resource Group

Other complete protein vegetarian sources include spirulina, hemp seed, amaranth and buckwheat.

Plant foods (which include fruits, vegetables, grains, nuts, legumes and seeds) do not provide all of the essential amino acids. They are called <u>incomplete proteins</u> or <u>low biological value proteins</u>. HOWEVER, vegetarians need not be dismayed.

Two incomplete proteins, eaten over the course of a day, can help form a complete protein. They are called <u>complementary proteins</u>. [38]

Great combinations for complementary proteins include eating legumes with grains, nuts or seeds. Remember, these do not have to be eaten together; they just need to be eaten over the course of each day. But here are some combinations in case you were curious: [38]

- Beans with rice or corn
- Beans and grains
- Hummus and pita bread
- Peanut butter on whole grain bread
- Pasta with beans
- Veggie burgers on bread

- Peanut butter and jelly sandwich
- Split pea soup with whole grain bread
- Tortillas and refried beans
- Lentil soup with cornbread
- Whole grain cereal with milk

Common Sources of Incomplete Proteins

Source	Portion Size	Grams of Protein
Pinto beans	½ cup (handful size)	11 grams
Chickpeas	½ cup	7 grams
Lentils	½ cup	9 grams
Edamame	½ cup	9 grams
Peas, green	½ cup	4 grams
Spinach, cooked	½ cup	3 grams
Peanut butter	1 Tb (size of thumb)	7 grams
Peanuts	1 oz (small handful)	7 grams
Sunflower seeds	1 oz (small handful)	6 grams

Table 13: Adapted from: Today's Dietitian

Chapter 7

Macronutrients: Carbohydrates

Carbohydrates

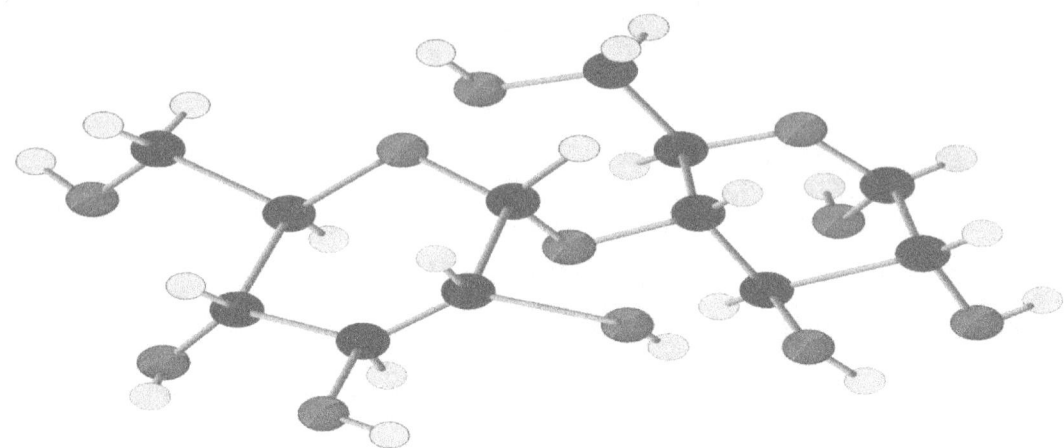

Disaccharide-Maltose

Put simply, carbohydrates provide <u>energy for your body.</u> They are also <u>part of DNA and RNA.</u> Carbohydrates include sugars, starches and fiber. [39]

There are 2 types: <u>simple carbohydrates</u> and <u>complex carbohydrates</u>. [39] Depending on the type depends on how quickly it is broken down in the body. The larger the carbohydrate, as in complex carbohydrates, the longer it takes the body to break it down, which is good news: you feel fuller longer!

Simple carbohydrates, also called simple sugars, are found naturally in foods such as fruits and milk. These provide ample vitamins and minerals and are important as part of a healthy lifestyle routine.

Simple carbohydrates are also found in refined sugars such as candy, regular sodas, syrups and table sugar. Let's keep the refined sugars intake to a minimum since they are considered empty calories. [39]

<u>Empty calories</u> provide little to no vitamins and minerals while, at the same time, causing excess intake of calories. AKA: eventual excess in body weight leading to overweight and obesity.

Monosaccharides are single sugars and include glucose, fructose, galactose and ribose. [40]

- Glucose is also called blood sugar. All carbohydrates are broken down into glucose, thus making glucose the main energy source for cells.
- Fructose is found in fruits.
- Galactose is found in milk.
- Ribose is part of RNA and deoxyribose is part of DNA.

Disaccharides are double sugars and include maltose, lactose and sucrose. They are two single sugars connected by a glycosidic bond and will break down into simple carbohydrates within the body. [40]

- Maltose is a glucose-glucose bond and is a malt sugar.
- Lactose is a glucose-galactose bond and is a milk sugar.
- Sucrose is a glucose-fructose bond and is found in table sugar.

Complex carbohydrates, also called complex sugars or polysaccharides, are long chains of monosaccharide sugars. According to the Food and Agriculture Organization (FAO), these are the foods that take longer to break down to simple sugars and, as a result, they delay gastric emptying and lead to quicker satiety. AKA: make you fill fuller for longer! [41]

Complex carbohydrates, or polysaccharides, are your starches and fibers that are found in plant foods. [42]

Starches are found in foods such as rice, grains products, corn, beans and potatoes. [43] Since they are large structures, it takes them longer to break down into simple sugars. One type of starch, resistant starch, has potentially great health benefits, but we'll talk about that when we talk about functional foods (which, by the way, is my FAV section. It really is, and it may end up being your favorite as well!).

Dietary fibers are the parts of the plant that do not break down entirely in the body. Fiber can be further classified as soluble and insoluble and each provides their own benefits to the body, such as <u>heart health</u>, <u>regulating the digestive tract</u> and helping you <u>feel fuller for longer</u>. [43] Fibers include foods such as beans, whole grains, brown rice, popcorn, nuts, berries, bran cereal, oatmeal and vegetables. [44] We'll discuss the types and sources of fiber in greater detail in the functional foods section.

Just for informational sake, let's take a deeper look at the sources, portion sizes and grams of carbohydrates.

Common Sources of Monosaccharides and Disaccharides

Source	Portion Size	Grams of Carbohydrate
Apple	1 medium	16 grams
Watermelon	1 (4"x8" wedge)	25 grams
Orange	1 medium	14 grams
Banana	1 medium	21 grams
Milk	1 cup	12 grams

Table 14: Adapted from: Nutrition Throughout the Lifecycle

This next list of simple sugars should be kept to a minimum because they are considered empty calories and provide mostly calories and sugar without the added benefits of vitamins and minerals that you would get from simple sugars such as fruits and milk.

Source	Portion size	Grams of Carbohydrate
Hard candy	1 oz	28 grams
Caramel	1 oz	21 grams
Fudge	1 oz	21 grams
Milk chocolate	1 oz	16 grams
Soda	12 oz	38 grams

Table 15: Adapted from: Nutrition Throughout the Lifecycle

Some cereals can be tricky as they can contain both simple and complex carbohydrates; sometimes naturally and sometimes through added sugars. Be on the lookout to avoid any added sugars such as molasses, corn sweetener, sucrose, lactose, glucose and high fructose corn syrup.

Common Sources of Polysaccharides

Source	Portion Size	Grams of Carbohydrate
Oatmeal	1/2 cup	12 grams
Whole wheat bread	1 slice	7 grams
White rice, cooked	1/2 cup	21 grams
Pasta, cooked	1/2 cup	15 grams
**Consume at least 1/2 of your grains as whole grains to get recommended amounts of fiber	(For example, brown rice, whole wheat bread, oatmeal, whole grain cereal, popcorn, whole wheat pasta)	
Lima beans	1/2 cup	11 grams
Kidney beans	1/2 cup	12 grams
Potato	1 medium	30 grams
Corn	1/2 cup	10 grams

Table 16: Adapted from: Nutrition Throughout the Lifecycle

Common Sources of Fiber

Source	Portion Size	Grams of Fiber
All Bran	1/2 cup	10 grams
Raisin Bran	1 cup	7 grams
Oatmeal	1 cup	4 grams
Whole wheat bread	1 slice	2 grams
Bran	2 Tb	2 grams
Avocado	1/2 medium	7 grams
Raspberries	1 cup	5 grams
Apple (with skin)	1 medium	3.3 grams
Banana	1 medium	3.1 grams
Strawberries	10 medium	2.1 grams
Potato (with skin)	1 medium	3.5 grams
Brussels sprouts	1/2 cup	3 grams
Broccoli	1/2 cup	2.8 grams
Carrots	1/2 cup	2.8 grams
Cauliflower	1/2 cup	2.5 grams
Corn	1/2 cup	2 grams
Pinto beans	1/2 cup	10 grams
Lentils	1/2 cup	8 grams
Kidney beans	1/2 cup	6.9 grams
Black-eye peas	1/2 cup	5.3 grams

Table 17: Adapted from: Nutrition Throughout the Lifecycle

Chapter 8

Macronutrients: Fat and Cholesterol

Fat and Cholesterol

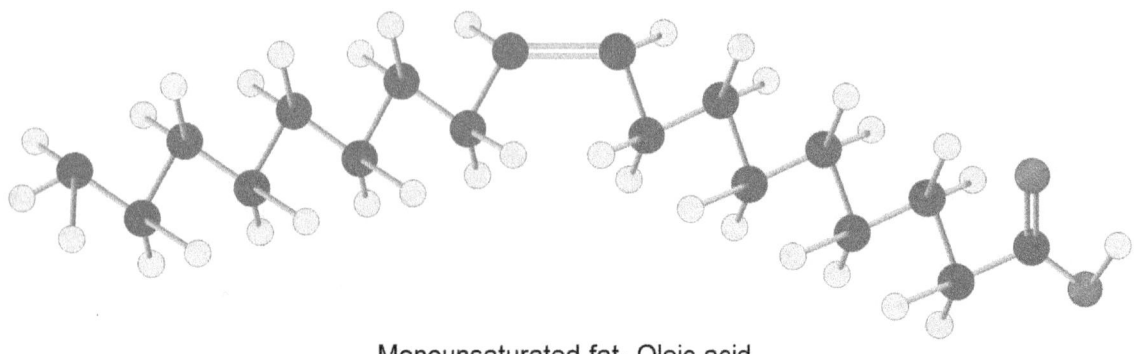

Monounsaturated fat- Oleic acid

Our bodies need fat for survival. [45] They are a source of concentrated energy and are <u>a part of cell membranes</u>. Fats help <u>carry fat soluble vitamins</u> through the body and they also are required for <u>normal growth and development</u>.

While fats are necessary for the body, they are not all created equally. I tend not to categorize any one food as "good" or "bad." When it comes to fats, though, there really are "good" and "bad" fats, so it is really important to pay attention to what kinds of fats provide the most benefits and which ones should be eaten sparingly.

Here are a few definitions from the American Heart Association (AHA) to start us off: [46]

<u>Low-density lipoprotein (LDL) cholesterol</u>-This is the bad cholesterol. It contributes to atherosclerosis (hardening of arteries) which can lead to a heart attack or stroke.

<u>High-density lipoprotein (HDL) cholesterol</u>- This is the good cholesterol and can help lower your risk of heart disease and stroke. The mechanism is as follows: HDL carries LDL to the liver where it is converted into bile. This bile is then excreted from the body as part of normal body processes. [47]

<u>Triglycerides</u>- This is the storage form of fat. An excess of calories will get converted into triglycerides and stored in the body. A prolonged excess of calories can lead to an increased formation of triglycerides, and thus eventual problems with overweight, obesity and atherosclerosis. [46]

The reason I wanted to give a few definitions is because the type of fat that we are about to discuss affects the levels of HDL, LDL and triglycerides.

I'll spout off a little chemistry here and there, but not much. I don't want to make myself cry again, haha.

Saturated Fats

Saturated fats raise the level of LDL cholesterol within your body, which, as we discussed earlier, is definitely not good and can lead to heart disease. Saturated fats should be kept to a minimum. [45]

Food sources of saturated fats include: [45]

Butter	Cream
Red meats	Lard
Whole milk	Cheese
Chicken with skin	

They can also be found in tropical oils such as: [45]

Palm oil	Cocoa butter
Coconut oil	

As you can see from the list, these food sources are solid at room temperature. This is because they only have single bonds which are saturated with hydrogen atoms. This allows them to wrap around easily and pack closely together forming a solid.

Trans Fats

These are the worst because not only do they raise the level of bad LDL cholesterol, they also lower the level of good HDL cholesterol, as reported by the AHA. A double yucky whammy for heart disease and stroke potential. [45]

While some trans fats are found naturally in animal products, the majority of trans fats in our diets comes from:

Baked goods such as: [45]

Cakes	Pie crusts
Biscuits	Cookies
Stick margarine	

Snacks such as: [45]

Potato chips	Some butter flavored popcorn

Fried foods such as: [45]

Some donuts	Fried chicken
French fries	

Some chain fast food restaurants, such as Chick-fil-A® and McDonald's®, have started to cut out the trans fats in their French fries.

Trans fats are created through processing. Yep, that word processed foods. If you take a vegetable oil (which we'll discuss later has multiple double bonds) and add hydrogen atoms, it becomes "partially hydrogenated oil", and less resistant to spoilage. And for those who care about the origins of a name, the original cis isomer of vegetable oil becomes a trans isomer, thus the term trans fat.

Who would think that one simple change can cause so much havoc in our body over time? Well, believe it, because it does. But there is some good news! The Food and Drug Administration (FDA) is requiring that all food manufacturers must stop using trans fats by July 2018. Most trans fat may be eliminated from our diets all together; woot! [49]

HOWEVER, too much of ANY fat over time can lead to overweight-, obesity- and health-related problems. And you still will want to watch your saturated fat intake.

Monounsaturated Fats

Monounsaturated fats are the bee's knees; they help lower LDL cholesterol levels AND raise HDL cholesterol levels, which helps reduce your risk of heart disease. Woot! [50]

You can find them in:[45]

Almonds	Avocados
Canola oil	Olive oil
Peanut oil	Safflower oil
Vegetable oil contains some polyunsaturated fats	

Monounsaturated fats are liquid at room temperature and only turn slightly solid when they are at refrigerator temperature. The reason for this is called stereochemistry. Monounsaturated fats have one (hence mono) double bond. This double bond causes a slight kink in the structure, which makes it hard to fold in around itself and, therefore, harder to form a solid. The unsaturated part comes from the fact that there are less hydrogen atoms saturating the structure.

Polyunsaturated Fats

Polyunsaturated fats are also extremely beneficial! They lower LDL cholesterol levels (Yay!), but at the same time, they also lower HDL cholesterol levels (boo). [50]

"Poly" means many and unsaturated, for this discussion, means unsaturated with hydrogen atoms. The less hydrogen atoms that are on the fat structure, the more double bonds that are there. As discussed earlier, these double bonds cause kinks and since there are multiple double bonds on polyunsaturated fats, they are completely liquid.

Have you heard a lot of talk about omega-3 and omega-6 fats? Well, those are found in polyunsaturated fats and are considered essential fatty acids. What that means is that your body will not synthesize them, so they must be obtained through food. You'll want to make sure you get your omega-3 and omega-6's because they are vital for brain function and cell growth, according to the National Library of Medicine (NLM). [51]

Omega-3 and omega-6 differ in chemical structure only by where the placement of the first double bond is. It is between the 6th and 7th carbon atom from the methyl end on the omega-6 and between the 3rd and 4th carbon atom from the methyl end on the omega-3. That's all I'll say about that because, quite frankly, I think we've been doing a lot of fat talk and it is extremely detailed already without adding chemical structure.

Some food sources of omega-3 fatty acids are: [52]

Walnuts	Flaxseed oil
Canola oil (also contains monounsaturated fats)	Tofu
Fish	Soybeans

 Side note: Omega-3's contain docosahexaenoic acid (DHA) and eicosapentaenoic acid (EPA). These have really amazing health benefits as well, but we'll talk about that in the functional foods section. Boom. Cliff hanger!

Some food sources of omega-6 fatty acids are: [52]

Vegetable oil	Corn oil
Safflower oil (also contains monounsaturated fats)	Soybean oil (also contains omega 3's)
Animal fats	

Most Americans have a high omega-6 to omega-3 ratio. That means we are consuming too many omega-6 fats and not enough omega-3 fats. Excessive omega-6 can lead to heart disease and other health diseases. [53]

So this is the gist:

The fat ranking from most beneficial to least beneficial is:
1) Monounsaturated fats (think avocado, olive oil, almonds)
2) Omega-3 polyunsaturated fat   (think walnuts, flaxseed oil, canola oil, fish)
3) Omega-6 polyunsaturated fat   (think vegetable oil)
4) Saturated fats (think animal fats like whole milk and red meat)
5) Trans-fatty acids   (think certain baked goods, processed foods, fried foods and some snack foods)

Let's take a look at those food sources again, some serving sizes and grams of fat just for information sake.

Common Sources of Saturated Fats

Source	Portion Size	Grams of Saturated Fats
Margarine	1 tsp	2.9 grams
Butter	1 tsp	2.4 grams
Salad dressing	1 Tb	1.2 grams
Cheddar cheese	1 oz	5.9 grams
American cheese	1 oz	5.5 grams
Cottage cheese	1/2 cup	3 grams
Milk, whole	1 cup	2.9 grams
Hamburger, 21% fat	3 oz	6.7 grams
Sausage, links	4	5.6 grams
Hot dog	1	4.9 grams
Chicken, fried, with skin	3 oz	3.8 grams
Salami	3 oz	3.6 grams
Croissant with egg, bacon, cheese	1	16 grams
Cheeseburger	1	9 grams

Table 17: Adapted from: Nutrition Throughout the Lifecycle

Common sources of Unsaturated Fats

Source	Portion Size	Grams of Unsaturated Fats
Hamburger, 21% fat	3 oz	10.9 grams (also has saturated fats so moderation)
Haddock	3 oz	6.5 grams
Chicken, baked, no skin	3 oz	6 grams
Pork chop, lean	3 oz	5.3 grams
Egg	1	5 grams
Sunflower seeds	1 oz	16.6 grams
Almonds	1 oz	12.6 grams
Peanuts	1 oz	11.3 grams
Cashews	1 oz	10.2 grams

Table 18: Adapted from: Nutrition Throughout the Lifecycle

Common Sources of Omega 3 Fatty Acids

Source	Portion Size	EPA and DHA Milligrams
Fish oil	1 tsp	2796 mg
Salmon, farmed	3 oz	1825 mg
Whitefish	3 oz	1370 mg
Mackerel	3 oz	1023 mg
Sardines	3 oz	840 mg
Flounder	3 oz	426 mg
Trout, freshwater	3 oz	420 grams
Oysters	3 oz	375 grams
Snapper	3 oz	273 grams
Shrimp	3 oz	268 grams
Catfish, wild	3 oz	201 grams
Crawfish	3 oz	187 grams
Tuna, light, in oil	3 oz	109 grams
DHA fortified egg	1	150 grams
Breastmilk	4 oz	126 grams

Table 19: Adapted from: Nutrition Throughout the Lifecycle

Chapter 9

Acceptable Macronutrient Range and Related Calculations

*The following grams, percentages and calculations are purely informational. I am not asking you to keep track of every bite of food you take and every gram it consists of and then translate it to a percentage, etc.

Acceptable Macronutrient Distribution Range

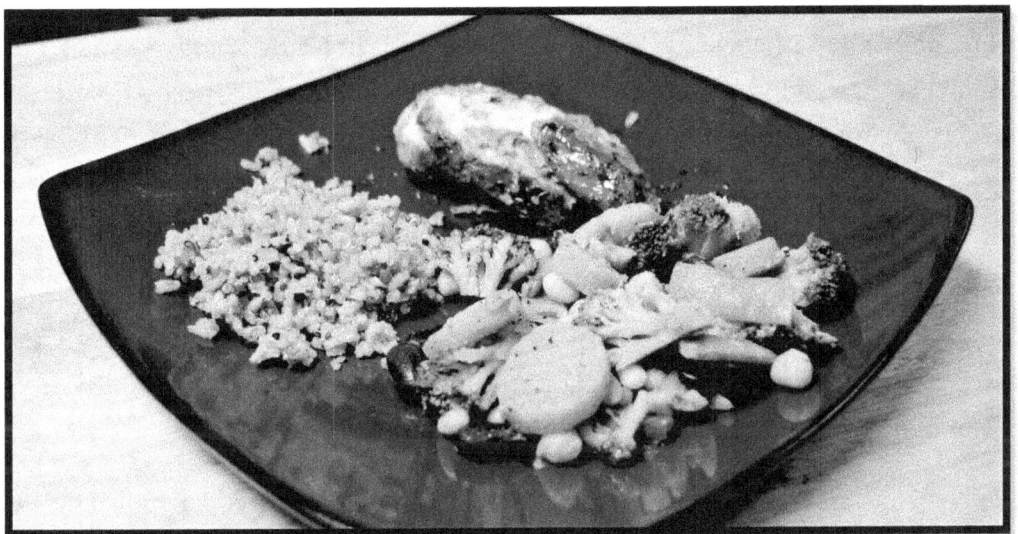

In the last few chapters, we looked at food sources, serving sizes and grams for each macronutrient. Let's figure out how those translate to your life.

Let's start with protein. There are high protein diets out there, but the Best Method is to eat a variety and balance of foods in order to obtain all the necessary nutrients that your body requires for health. That is where the Acceptable Macronutrient Distribution Range (AMDR), from the National Academies of Sciences (NAS), comes in. [54]

The protein AMDR for adults is 10-35%.

This means that 10-35% of your food intake, through calories, should come through protein. A consistent deficiency in protein can mean your body is not getting the required protein to build muscle and activate chemical reactions. A consistent excess can mean that you are lacking in other macronutrients, such as fat and carbohydrates, which are also vital to your health. We'll talk about that, along with some percent-to-gram-to-calorie calculations in a little while.

The carbohydrate AMDR for adults is 45-65%.

A consistent deficiency in carbohydrates can lead to malnutrition and a consistent excess can lead to overweight and obesity. Remember, the key is balance. Too little or too much of anything on this planet can break up homeostasis and eventually lead to imbalance.

The fat AMDR for adults is 20-35% with 5-10% coming from omega-6 and .6-1.2% coming from omega-3.

As discussed earlier, your body needs fat for survival. However, keep in mind that you want to choose the healthy fats most of the time for optimal health.

But what does that mean to me, you might be asking? For most, it just highlights the need for balance of all macronutrients in order to maintain long-term balance within your body. For some, they may like to take those percentages and convert them to grams and calories, and I'll show you how to do that. But, again, I am not expecting you to count calories, grams or percentages. It's just good-to-know information in case you get more in-depth in the future with your health goals. For example, if you have lost the weight and now want to start really lifting weights for muscle building, this can help you figure out your optimal protein level maximum and how to fit it into your daily routine.

We figured out the AMDR for our macronutrients are:

Protein: 10-35%
Carbohydrate: 45-65%
Fat: 20-35%

Remember the chart in the first chapter that listed your calorie needs per day? Please pull that number back out again or you can just look it up again here if you need:

Daily Caloric Intake Needs

Activity Level Age	MALE			FEMALE		
	Sedentary	Moderately Active	Active	Sedentary	Moderately Active	Active
2	1,000	1000	1000	1000	1000	1000
3	1200	1400	1400	1000	1200	1400
4	1200	1400	1600	1200	1400	1400
5	1200	1400	1600	1200	1400	1600
6	1400	1600	1800	1200	1400	1600
7	1400	1600	1800	1200	1600	1800
8	1400	1600	2000	1400	1600	1800
9	1600	1800	2000	1400	1600	1800
10	1600	1800	2200	1400	1800	2000
11	1800	2000	2200	1600	1800	2000
12	1800	2200	2400	1600	2000	2200
13	2000	2200	2600	1600	2000	2200
14	2000	2400	2800	1800	2000	2400
15	2200	2600	3000	1800	2000	2400
16	2400	2800	3200	1800	2000	2400
17	2400	2800	3200	1800	2000	2400
18	2400	2800	3200	1800	2000	2400
19-20	2600	2800	3000	2000	2200	2400
21-25	2400	2800	3000	2000	2000	2400
26-30	2400	2600	3000	1800	2000	2400
31-35	2400	2600	3000	1800	2000	2200
36-40	2400	2600	2800	1800	2000	2200
41-45	2200	2600	2800	1800	2000	2200
46-50	2200	2400	2800	1800	2000	2200
51-55	2200	2400	2800	1600	1800	2200
56-60	2200	2400	2600	1600	1800	2200
61-65	2000	2400	2600	1600	1800	2000
66-70	2000	2200	2600	1600	1800	2000
71-75	2000	2200	2600	1600	1800	2000
76+	2000	2200	2400	1600	1800	2000

Table 2: Adapted from: Center for Nutrition Policy and Promotion, USDA

Sedentary- light physical activity involving day-to-day activities

Moderately active- equivalent of walking 1.5-3 miles per day along with day-to-day activities

Active- equivalent of walking more than 3 miles per day along with day-to-day activities

Calculations

Calculate calories needed from each macronutrient using the AMDR

> The most typical daily goal for macronutrient consumption is 60% carbohydrate, 30% fat and 10% protein.

Let's say you need 2,200 calories per day for a 55 year old male, sedentary, 205 pounds, 5'9"

- 2,200 calories x .60 = 1320 calories from carbohydrates each day.
- 2,200 calories x .30 = 660 calories from fat each day.
- 2,200 calories x .10 = 220 calories from protein each day.

Calculate grams per macronutrient based on calories [55]

> There are 4 calories per gram of protein.
> There are 4 calories per gram of carbohydrate.
> There are 9 calories per gram of fat.
> There are 7 calories per gram of alcohol. We won't be using this one, but it's a good-to-know kind of thing.

As established above, this male will need 1,320 calories from carbohydrate, 660 calories from fat and 220 calories from protein each day.

Let's translate that to grams.

- 1,320 carbohydrate calories divided by 4 = 330 grams carbohydrate needed each day.
- 660 fat calories divided by 9 = 73.3 grams of fat needed each day.
- 220 protein calories divided by 4 = 55 grams of protein needed each day.

And voila'! You have converted total calories needed into percentages needed into calories per macronutrient into grams. Whew.

You can use the conversions back and forth depending on what information you're working with.

Calculate calories per macronutrient based on grams

___ grams of carbohydrate listed on nutrition label package x 4 calories per gram = ____ total calories from carbohydrate.

____ grams of protein listed on nutrition label package x 4 calories per gram = ___ total calories from protein.

____ grams of fat listed on nutrition label package x 9 calories per gram = ____ total calories from fat.

Calculate percentage of total calories from each macronutrient

____ calories from carbohydrates in food item divided by ____ total calories in food item x 100 = ____ % from carbohydrates.

____ calories from protein in food item divided by _____ total calories in food item x 100 = ____ % from protein.

____ calories from fat in food item divided by _____ total calories in food item x 100 = ____% from fat.

Okay, enough of that. Let's move on, shall we?

Chapter 10

Fluids

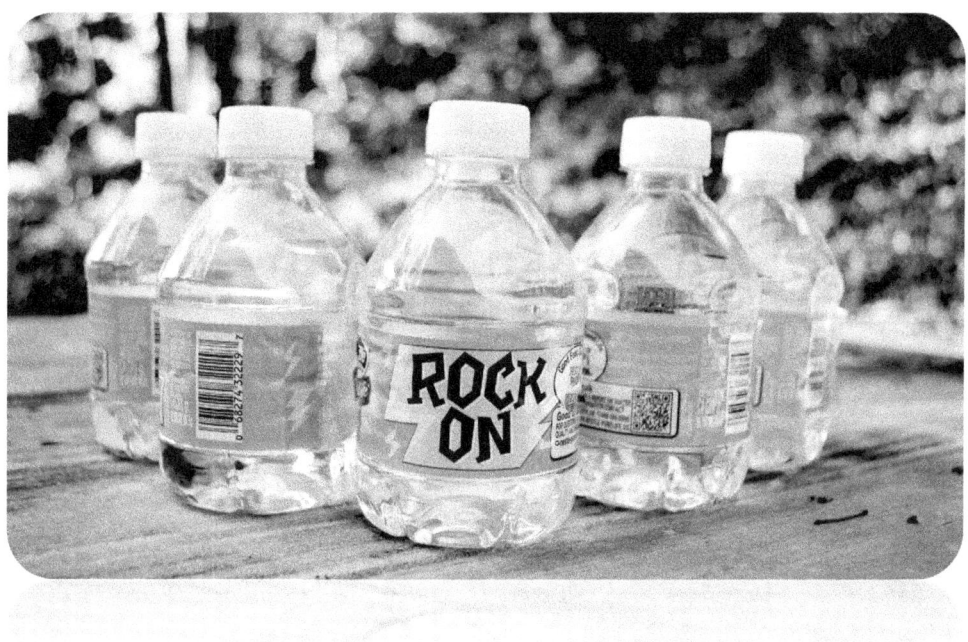

Who can forget about water?

You can live up to 60 days without food (as long as water is provided), but only 3 days without water, states *Nutrition Through the Life Cycle.* [56]

That's because water is vital to our survival. Water helps <u>regulate temperature</u>, <u>transport nutrients</u> and <u>remove waste</u> from our body. [57]

Drinking too much water can lead to heart and kidney failure. Drinking too little water can lead to dehydration, headache, dry mouth, dizziness, muscle spasms and eventual kidney failure. Again, moderation and balance.

The **Adequate Intake** for fluids is 11 cups per day for women and 15 cups per day for men, according to NAS. [58]

What?? That's insane. Well, the good news is that it is talking about FLUIDS, not just straight up water from your bottle or glass.

There are multiple ways that fluids count towards your total intake, such as through food and almost all beverages except alcohol.

For example:

> Food intake accounts for approximately 20% of your fluid intake. [59]

So let's go ahead and subtract that from the huge 11 cups for women and 15 cups for men.

Remember, each cup is about the size of your fist.

> Women: 11 cups x .20 = 2.2   11 cups – 2.2 = 8.8
>
> -   8.8 cups of beverages needed each day for women
>
> Men: 15 cups x .20 = 3   15 cups – 3 = 12
>
> -   12 cups of beverages needed each day for men

That still sounds crazy. But, again, we're talking about fluids, not just water. The beverages each day can include: [58]

Tea   Coffee   Juice   Soda   Drinking water

Some of the beverages listed contain caffeine. Caffeine is a stimulant that has a laxative effect and increases urine production, so it seems that those would not count towards total fluid intake sources. [59] However, they do count since their consumption does not contribute to greater dehydration. [59]

Also, we will not count alcohol into the beverage category because drinking more than 1 drink for women per day and 2 drinks for men per day can have negative health effects. So we'll just leave that one out for this discussion.

What are some ways you can think of to drink more fluids without the excess calories?

_____

_____

Maybe you can carry around a tumbler of ice water and add a bag of green tea in it for 15 minutes for a nice cold-brewed tea. Or maybe prepare and keep some unsweetened iced tea in the refrigerator and drink it throughout the week. And some just really love the taste of ice cold refreshing water all by itself!

It is important to note that if you are physically active or live in a hot or humid area, you will need more fluids. [58]

Let's look at another way to figure out daily fluids needed if you know approximately how many calories you consume each day: [60]

Most people need 1 mL per calorie consumed.
Let's say you consume 2,200 calories per day.
That would be 2,200 calories = 2,200 mL of fluids needed each day.
1 cup = 237 mL
2,200 mL divided by 237 = 9.28 cups per day of fluids

If you are not sure how many calories you consume each day, then here is another equation.

Most people need 30 mL per kg of weight each day in fluid. [61] Just bear with me again with the metric conversions, please.

Conversions to kg:

Weight: 1 kg = 2.2 lb   Weight in pounds_____ divided by 2.2 = _____ kg

---

Weight in kilograms x 30 mL = daily fluid requirement

For example: Male, 205 pounds:

---

205 lb divided by 2.2 = 93.18 kilograms

93.18 kg x 30 mL = 2795.4 mL per day

2795.4 mL divided by 237 = 11.8 cups   (1 cup = 237 mL)

On to the micronutrients!

Chapter 11

Micronutrients: Vitamins

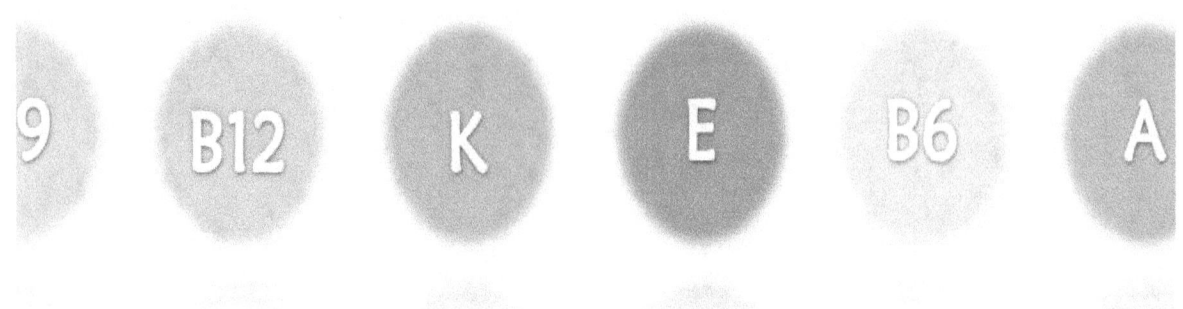

Since there is so much information for vitamins and minerals, I'd like to break things up a bit. So after each of the vitamin and mineral discussions, we'll do a few fun activities. Maybe that will also help us retain the information a little better!

Micronutrients (vitamins and minerals) are not required in large amounts; hence the word micro in the name. [62] However, not getting enough micronutrients can have devastating effects on health. For example, a mother not ingesting enough folic acid during pregnancy can lead to neural tube defects for her child.

Getting too much of a particular vitamin or mineral can be detrimental to your health as well. For example, too much Vitamin A can lead to nausea, dry skin, liver damage and birth defects.

Dare I say it? Balance. Moderation. Eating a variety of foods from the food groups can help with that balance.

Most vitamins and minerals MUST be supplied by our diet. With the exception of Vitamin D (with the help of sunlight) and Vitamin K, the body does not produce vitamins and minerals on its own. [62]

Let's start with vitamins.[63]

When it comes to vitamins, there are fat-soluble and water-soluble. [63]

Fat-soluble vitamins are absorbed in fat and those fats transport them throughout the body. Since fat is stored in our bodies, it is possible to accumulate too many fat-soluble vitamins, which can lead to toxicity. [64]

The fat-soluble vitamins are DEKA: Vitamin D, Vitamin E, Vitamin K and Vitamin A.

Water-soluble vitamins are absorbed in water and water transports them throughout the body. A person is less likely to have a toxicity of water-soluble vitamins since water is constantly being taken in and excreted each day. However, an overabundance of any micronutrient may lead to health problems. Since water-soluble vitamins are constantly moving with the water in and out of our bodies, we need a more consistent supply.[63]

These include vitamins such as Vitamin B1 (thiamine), B2 (riboflavin), B3 (niacin), B5 (pantothenic acid), B6 (pyroxidine), B7 (biotin), B9 (folate), B12 (cobalamin) and Vitamin C.

Fat-Soluble Vitamins: DEKA

Vitamin D	
Functions	
-Enhances calcium absorption to help build and maintain healthy teeth and bones -Helps immune system, brain, nervous system, skin, muscles, cartilage, reproductive organs and red blood cells	-Helps regulate blood pressure -May help prevent certain cancers
Deficiency	
-Rickets Rickets- softening and weakening of bones	-Osteoporosis
Toxicity	
-Abnormal high blood calcium -Stunted growth	-Vomiting
Good sources	
-Sunlight -Fortified milk -Eggs	-Fortified cereals -Fatty fish -Liver

Table 21: Adapted from: Food and Agriculture Organization and Food and Nutrition Service

Fortified- nutrients added to foods or drinks that were not originally in the food or drink.

Enriched- nutrients that were lost during processing and were added back to the food or drink.

Vitamin E	
Functions	
-Helps form red blood cells, muscles and other tissues	-May help reduce risk of heart disease
-Antioxidant which may help protect against certain cancers	
(We'll learn more about antioxidants in the next chapter; my favorite chapter!)	
Deficiency	
-Newborn hemolytic anemia	-Retinal degeneration
Anemia- low count of healthy red blood cells	
Toxicity	
-May interfere with Vitamin K, so prolonged clotting time	
Good sources	
-Vegetable oil	-Green leafy vegetables
-Liver	-Whole grains
-Egg yolk	-Fortified or enriched cereals
-Butter	

Table 22: Adapted from: Food and Agriculture Organization and Food and Nutrition Service

Vitamin K	
Functions	
-Assists in blood clotting	-Synthesis by intestinal bacteria
-Needed for bone formation	
Deficiency	
-Prolonged bleeding	-Hemorrhage in newborns
Toxicity	
-Hemolytic anemia	-Jaundice
	Jaundice- yellowing of the skin; visible sign of a potential disease or problem
Good sources	
-Vegetable oil	-Pork
-Green leafy vegetables	-Liver

Table 23: Adapted from: Food and Agriculture Organization and Food and Nutrition Service

Vitamin A	
Functions	
-Essential for eyesight, skin, reproduction, growth, respiratory tissue and digestive tract tissue -Proper function of immune system and fighting infection	-Growth and reproduction of hair, bones and teeth -May help protect against certain cancers (as beta carotene- precursor of Vit A providing red orange, yellow pigments in fruit, vegetables)
Deficiency	
-Night blindness -Poor bone growth	-Impaired resistance to infection
Toxicity	
-Fatigue -Night sweats -Headache -Stunted growth	-Bone pain -Vomiting -Jaundice
Good sources	
-Liver -Egg yolk	-Deep yellow and orange vegetables -Dark green vegetables

Table 24: Adapted from: Food and Agriculture Organization and Food and Nutrition Service

Water-Soluble Vitamins (Vitamin B1, B2, B3, B5, B6, B7, B9, B12 and Vitamin C)

Vitamin B$_1$ (Thiamine)	
Functions	
-Necessary for carbohydrate metabolism	-Promotes healthy nerve function
-Needed for muscular, cardiovascular, nervous and gastrointestinal systems	
Deficiency	
-Edema	-Cardiac failure
Toxicity	
N/A	
Good sources	
-Lean pork	-Enriched breads and cereal
-Wheat germ	-Legumes
-Whole grains	-Potatoes

Table 25: Adapted from: Food and Agriculture Organization and Food and Nutrition Service

Vitamin B$_2$ (Riboflavin)	
Functions	
-Essential for growth	-Helps release energy to cells
-Necessary for metabolism of foods	-Essential for proper B6 and B3 function
Deficiency	
-Poor growth	
Toxicity	
N/A	
Good sources	
-Meat	-Green vegetables
-Dairy products	-Whole grains
-Egg yolk	-Fortified and enriched grains
-Legumes	

Table 26: Adapted from: Food and Agriculture Organization and Food and Nutrition Service

B₃ (Niacin)	
Functions	
-Helps enzymes convert food into energy	-Maintains healthy digestive tract, nervous system and skin
Deficiency	
-Dermatitis	-Dementia
-Diarrhea	
Toxicity	
-Tingling sensation	-Nausea
-Dizziness	
Good sources	
-Meat	Whole grains
-Poultry	-Enriched grains
-Fish	-Egg yolk

Table 27: Adapted from: Food and Agriculture Organization and Food and Nutrition Service

B₅ (Pantothenic acid)	
Functions	
-Energy metabolism	-Formation of hormones and chemicals for nerve function
Deficiency	
-Fatigue	-Muscle cramps
-Sleep disturbance	-Loss of antibody production
-Nausea	
Toxicity	
-Diarrhea	-Water retention
Good sources	
-Meat	-Egg yolk
-Fish	-Whole grains
-Poultry	-Legumes
-Liver	-Vegetables

Table 28: Adapted from: Food and Agriculture Organization and Food and Nutrition Service

B$_6$ (Pyridoxine)	
Functions	
-Absorption and metabolism of protein	-Nerve and brain function
-Absorption of carbohydrates	-Helps make protein in the body
-Helps form blood cells	
Deficiency	
-Microcytic anemia	-Irritability
<u>Anemia</u>- low count of healthy red blood cells	
-Convulsions	
Toxicity	
-Photosensitivity	-Bone pain
Good sources	
-Liver	-Legumes
-Meat	-Potatoes
-Whole grains	

Table 29: Adapted from: Food and Agriculture Organization and Food and Nutrition Service

B7 (Biotin)	
Functions	
-Metabolism of carbohydrates, fats and proteins	-Essential for enzymes
Deficiency	
-Dermatitis	-Insomnia
-Nausea	-Depression
Toxicity	
N/A	
Good sources	
-Liver	-Most vegetables
-Meat	-Strawberries
-Egg yolk	-Grapefruit
-Yeast	-Watermelon
-Bananas	

Table 30: Adapted from: Food and Agriculture Organization and Food and Nutrition Service

B9 Folate (Folic acid)	*Folate is the natural form. *Folic acid is the synthetic form.
Functions	
-Production and maintenance of red blood cells	-Prevention of birth defects during pregnancy
Deficiency	
-Birth defects	-Megaloblastic anemia
-Poor growth	<u>Anemia</u>- low count of healthy red blood cells
-Impaired cell immunity	
Toxicity	
N/A	
Good sources	
-Liver	-Legumes
-Green leafy vegetables	-Oranges
-Legumes	-Cantaloupe
-Whole grains	-Lean beef
-Fortified or enriched grains	

Table 31: Adapted from: Food and Agriculture Organization and Food and Nutrition Service

B$_{12}$ (Cobalamin)	*Vegetarians may require supplementation.
Functions	
-Helps form new blood cells	-Healthy nervous system
Deficiency	
-Pernicious anemia	-Neurologic deterioration
Anemia- low count of healthy red blood cells	
Toxicity	
N/A	
Good sources	
-Meat	-Egg
-Fish	-Yolk
-Poultry	-Liver
-Cheese	

Table 32: Adapted from: Food and Agriculture Organization and Food and Nutrition Service

Vitamin C (Ascorbic acid)	
Functions	
-Collagen synthesis -Binds tissues and cells together -Healthy gums	-Antioxidant for cell protection -Improves wound healing and resistance to infection -Helps absorb iron in plant foods
Deficiency	
-Scurvy Scurvy- disease that causes weakness, anemia, gum disease and skin hemorrhages	-Hemorrhages -Bleeding gums
Toxicity	
-Nausea -Abdominal cramps	-Possible kidney stones
Good sources	
-Citrus fruits (papaya, cantaloupe, strawberries) -Potatoes	-Cabbage

Table 33: Adapted from: Food and Agriculture Organization and Food and Nutrition Service

I know reading tables can sometimes cause us to zone out, so, as I mentioned before, I wanted to make a few fun activities that will highlight some key ideas using everything from this chapter. I'll do the same for minerals.

Matching Game   Draw a line to the appropriate answer.

Citrus fruits

Anemia

Folate

Antioxidants

Vitamin D

Body tissues

Vitamin K

Fat

Rickets

Folic acid

Scurvy

Vegetarians

1) Vitamin E, Beta carotene and Vitamin C are vitamins that act as _____.

2) This is vitamin can be produced in the gut by intestinal bacteria.

3) _____ may need a B 12 vitamin and Vitamin D supplement (as well as minerals iron and calcium).

4) A deficiency in Vitamin C may lead to a disease called _____, which causes gum disease and skin hemorrhages.

5) A deficiency of Vitamin B12 or folate can cause _____ (mineral iron deficiency can also cause this).

6) Vitamins D, E, K, A are ___ soluble vitamins.

7) This vitamin can help prevent birth defects, such as spina bifida.

8) This vitamin enhances calcium absorption to help build and maintain strong bones and teeth.

9) These foods are a great source of Vitamin C.

10) A deficiency of Vitamin D (and also minerals calcium and phosphorus) can lead to this disorder which causes a softening and weakening of bones.

11) Toxicity is more likely in fat soluble vitamins because they can be stored in ____ _____.

12) _____ ____ is the synthetic form of folate.

*Answers are below crossword puzzle game

Crossword Puzzle

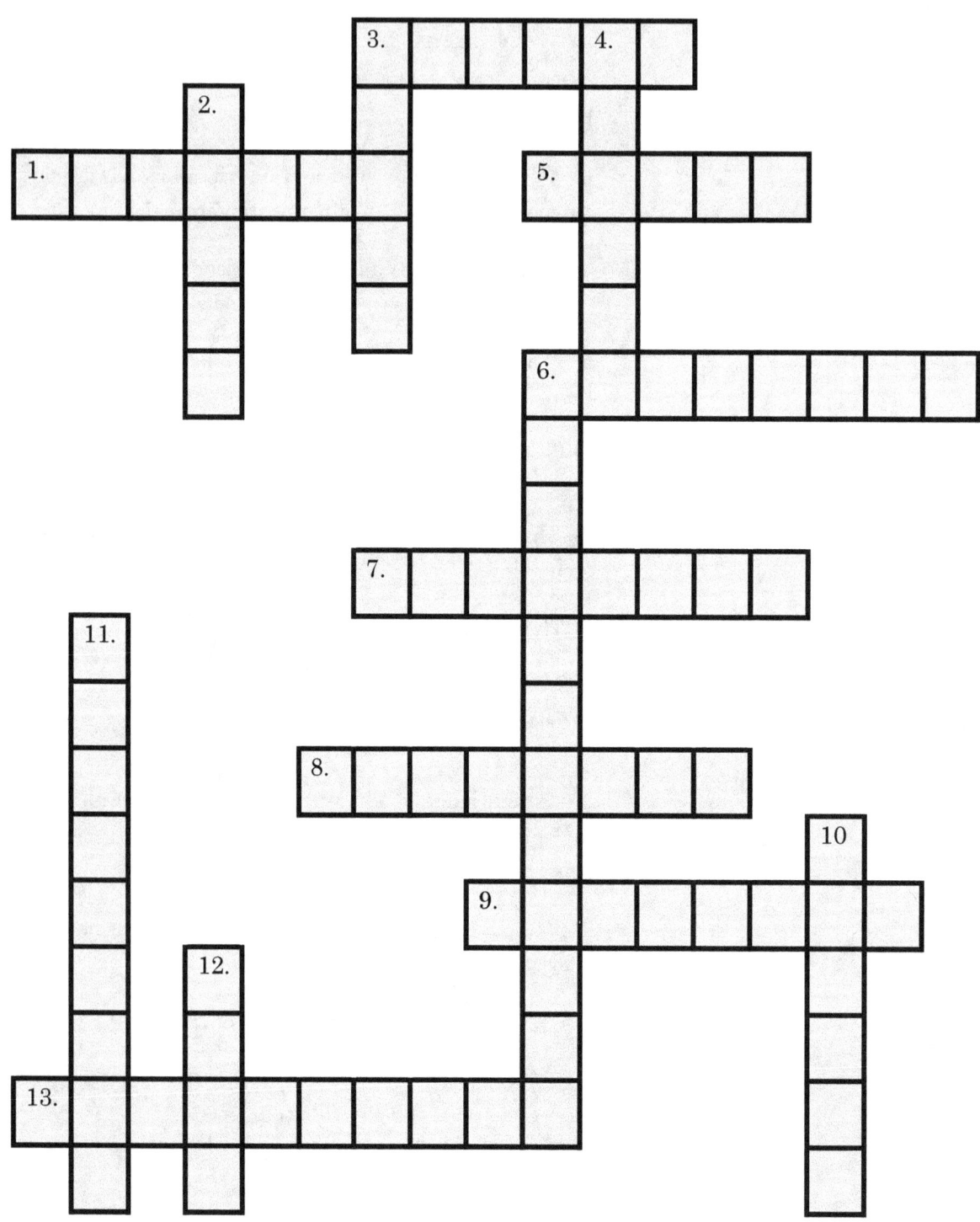

1) Vitamin C helps with improved wound _____ and resistance to infection.

2) Vitamin K assists in _____ clotting.

3 across) B Vitamins convert food into _____ throughout the day.

3 down) B-complex includes how many _____ vitamins (number).

4) A great food source for Vitamin E and B vitamins are whole _____.

5) A person is less likely to have toxicity of _____ soluble vitamins.

6 across) Another term for Vitamin C is _____ acid.

6 down) Vitamin C and Vitamin E act as _____ to help prevent cancer.

7) Nutrients that were lost during processing and added back in are called _____ nutrients.

8) _____ and milk are good sources of Vitamin D.

9) Beta _____ is the precursor of Vitamin A and acts as an antioxidant.

10) Vitamin B12 is naturally found in _____ products.

11) _____ nutrients are added to foods and drinks that were not originally contained in the food or drink.

12) With the exception of Vitamin D and Vitamin K, vitamins and minerals must be obtained through the ____.

13) A diet high in whole grains, _____, fruit, lean meats and dairy helps ensure adequate amounts of vitamins and minerals.

Key for matching game:

1) Antioxidants
2) Vitamin K
3) Vegetarians
4) Scurvy
5) Anemia
6) Fat
7) Folate
8) Vitamin D
9) Citrus fruits
10) Rickets
11) Body tissues
12) Folic acid

Key for crossword puzzle:

1) Healing
2) Blood
3) Energy
4) Eight
5) Grains
6) Water
7) Ascorbic
8) Antioxidant
9) Enriched
10) Sunlight
11) Carotene
12) Animal
13) Fortified
14) Diet
15) Vegetables

I am not going to lie, all this talk of healthy foods and health benefits just prompted me to make and eat a HUGE salad. I made sure to make enough to last a few days. Romaine, kale, tomatoes, cucumber, red onion, shredded carrots, mushrooms. Basically any vegetable in the refrigerator went into this salad... yum yum yum!

And who can forget the dressing? Consider dressings that add to your arsenal of health, such as olive oil/vinegar emulsions (such as some vinaigrettes).

My mother-in-law was kind enough to share her balsamic vinaigrette dressing. She never measures, so I did my best variation using her ingredients. Please feel free to add a little more or a little less of an ingredient depending on taste preference. It is so yummy; it will make you crave salad! And it tastes even better as the flavors meld overnight!

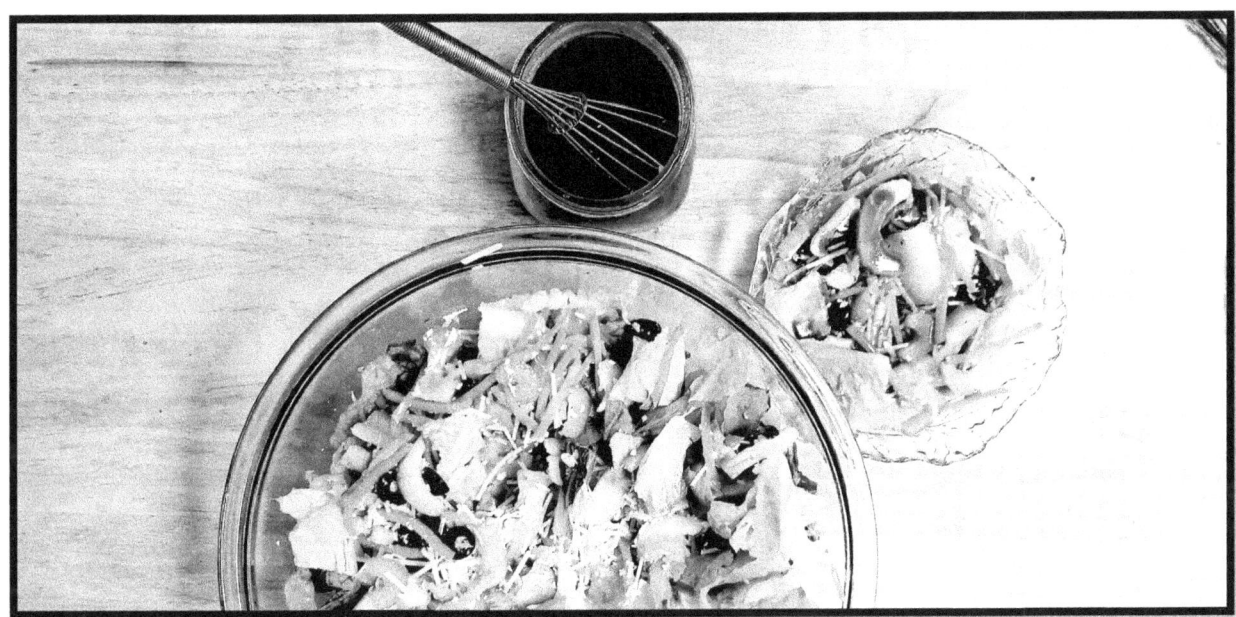

Balsamic Vinaigrette Dressing

2/3 cup olive oil

1/3 cup balsamic vinegar

2 cloves garlic, finely minced

2 Tbsp Dijon mustard (or more to taste)

2 Tbsp honey

1/2 tsp Worcestershire®

1/2 tsp hot sauce

1/4 tsp salt

1/4 tsp pepper

1) Whisk all ingredients together very well.
2) Pour into a mason jar with lid (or any container that has a tight seal).
3) Keep unused dressing in the refrigerator.

This particular salad dressing contains some potentially great nutrition benefits. We'll be talking more about these benefits in the functional foods chapter coming up next, but here's an example using this recipe:

- <u>Heart health</u> through monounsaturated fatty acids (olive oil), flavonols-catechins (vinegar) and diallyl sulfide/allyl methyl trisulfide (garlic).
- <u>Antibacterial effect</u> through flavonols-catechins (vinegar).
- <u>Reduced cancer risk</u> through inulin/oligosaccharides (honey), flavonols-quercetin (garlic), flavonols-catechins (vinegar) and selenium (garlic).
- <u>Digestive health</u> and <u>weight health</u> through inulin/oligosaccharides (honey, garlic).
- <u>Enhanced immunity</u> through diallyl sulfide/allyl methyl trisulfide (garlic).

And, oh my gosh, this is not even mentioning the antioxidants, vitamins, minerals and other healthity-health-health stuff in the salad!

Keep in mind, though, that while olive oil is a healthy fat, too much of any fat can add excessive and unnecessary calories. Luckily, this tangy-sweet vinaigrette is just right for lightly drizzling over a salad allowing it to bring out the freshness of both the dressing and the vegetables.

Side note: We had spaghetti last night and I made sure to add chopped spinach to the spaghetti, just to make things easier and healthier. And whole grain rolls on the side. Yummy!

Chapter 12

Micronutrients: Minerals

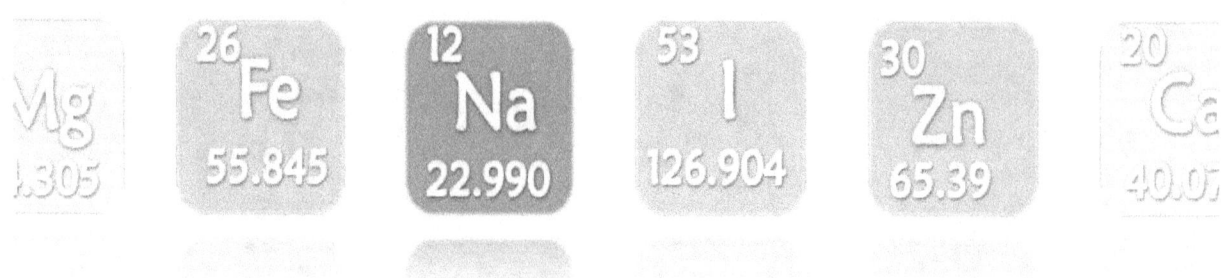

Similar to the chapter on vitamins, I would like to break things up a little after our mineral section and do a few activities. The goal of the activities is to allow us to get a more focused look at the information in the tables and it also helps to better learn the information.

Since vitamins and minerals are a micronutrient, they are only needed in micro amounts. As with vitamins, minerals are vital to our health. Getting too much or too little of a vitamin or mineral may have serious health consequences. However, eating a variety of protein, grains, dairy, fruits and vegetables helps keep our body in balance and helps avoid any natural deficiencies or toxicities.

Calcium
*Adequate calcium may help prevent osteoporosis. *Most American's are not getting enough calcium in their diets. [63]

Functions	
-Strong bones and teeth	-Helps convert food into energy
-Muscle and nerve function	-May help prevent high blood pressure

Deficiency
-Rickets
Rickets- abnormal formation of bones

Toxicity	
-Calcification of bones and soft tissue	-Lethargy
-Vomiting	

Good sources	
-Milk	-Tofu with calcium sulfate
-Yogurt	-Sardines
-Cheese	-Salmon
-Fortified or enriched grains	
-Some green leafy vegetables (collards, kale, turnip greens)	

Table 34: Adapted from: Food and Agriculture Organization and Food and Nutrition Service

Chloride	
Functions	
-Normal fluid balance	-Transport of carbon dioxide by blood cells
-Acid-base balance (electrolyte)	
(we'll talk more about electrolytes in the next chapter)	
Deficiency	
-Nausea	-Dizziness
-Cramps	-Apathy
-Vomiting	-Exhaustion
Toxicity	
-Vomiting	
Good sources	
-Table salt	

Table 35: Adapted from: Food and Agriculture Organization and Food and Nutrition Service

Chromium	
Functions	
-Metabolism of carbohydrate, protein and fat	-Helps with glucose metabolism
Deficiency	
-Glucose intolerance	-Impaired growth
Toxicity	
N/A	
Good sources	
-Meat	-Fortified or enriched grains
-Whole grains	-Corn oil

Table 36: Adapted from: Food and Agriculture Organization and Food and Nutrition Service

Cobalt	
Functions	
-Prevention of anemia -Helps with red blood cell production	-Healthy nervous system
Deficiency	
N/A	
Toxicity	
N/A	
Good sources	
N/A	

Table 37: Adapted from: Food and Agriculture Organization and Food and Nutrition Service

Copper	
Functions	
-Required for absorption and use of iron in making hemoglobin -Necessary for red blood cell formation, connective tissue and nerve fibers	-May help the immune system
Deficiency	
-Pallor Pallor- Pale skin appearance	
Toxicity	
-Copper deposition in cornea -Liver deterioration	-Deterioration of nerve processes
Good sources	
-Liver	-Shellfish
-Kidney	-Legumes
-Poultry	-Whole grains

Table 38: Adapted from: Food and Agriculture Organization and Food and Nutrition Service

Fluoride
Functions
-Resists acids and decay for healthy teeth   -Strong bones
Deficiency
-Increased tooth cavities
Toxicity
-Discolored teeth
Good sources
-Fluoridated water   -Toothpaste with fluoride

Table 39: Adapted from: Food and Agriculture Organization and Food and Nutrition Service

Iodine	
Functions	
-Helps form thyroid hormones	-Required for normal growth and functioning of brain and body
Deficiency	
-Goiter	-Cretinism
Goiter- abnormal enlargement of thyroid gland at the bottom of the neck.	Cretinism- underdeveloped physical and mental growth
Toxicity	
-Thyroid enlargement	
Good sources	
-Seafood	-Iodized salt

Table 40: Adapted from: Food and Agriculture Organization and Food and Nutrition Service

Iron
**Vegetarians may require supplementation.*
*Heme iron (from animals) is better absorbed than non-heme iron (from plant sources).

Functions	
-Transports oxygen throughout the body for energy production	-Helps immune system fight disease

Deficiency	
-Microcytic anemia	-Pallor
<u>Anemia</u>- low count of healthy red blood cells	-Lethargy
-Malabsorption	-Irritability

Toxicity	
-Liver disease	-Heart problems

Good sources	
-Red meat	-Whole grains
-Liver	-Fortified or enriched grains
-Clams, oysters	-Dark green vegetables
-Legumes	

Table 41: Food and Agriculture Organization and Food and Nutrition Service

Magnesium	
Functions	
-Necessary for genetic material	-Works with calcium for healthy bones and teeth
-Proper bone growth	
-Normal muscle and nerve function	-Helps regulate blood sugar levels
-Healthy immune system	-Helps normalize blood pressure
Deficiency	
-Muscle tremors	-Irritability
-Convulsions	
Toxicity	
-Diarrhea	
Good sources	
-Whole grains	-Legumes
-Tofu	-Green vegetables

Table 42: Food and Agriculture Organization and Food and Nutrition Service

Manganese	
Functions	
-Necessary for bone formation	-Helps metabolize protein, fat and carbohydrate
Deficiency	
-Impaired growth	-Skeletal abnormalities
Toxicity	
-Psychiatric and nerve disorders if high exposure	
Good sources	
-Whole grains	-Fruits
-Legumes	-Leafy vegetables

Table 43: Adapted from: Food and Agriculture Organization and Food and Nutrition Service

Molybdenum	
Functions	
-Helps with metabolism	-Regulation of iron storage
Deficiency	
-Rapid heartbeat	-Nausea and vomiting
Toxicity	
-Joint pain	-Growth failure
Good sources	
-Organ meats	-Dark green leafy vegetables
-Grains	-Legumes

Table 44: Adapted from: Food and Agriculture Organization and Food and Nutrition Service

Phosphorus	
Functions	
-Energy metabolism	-Transmission of DNA and RNA
-Necessary for growth	-Works with calcium for strong bones and teeth
-Nerve and muscle function	
Deficiency	
-Loss of appetite	-Loss of calcium from bones
-Weakness	
Toxicity	
-Muscle spasms	
Good sources	
-Cheese	-Fish
-Egg yolk	-Whole grains
-Beef, pork	-Legumes
-Poultry	

Table 45: Adapted from: Food and Agriculture Organization and Food and Nutrition Service

Potassium	
Functions	
-Acid-base balance	-Muscle contractions
-Fluid balance inside of cells	-Helps maintain regular heart rhythm
-Nerve impulses	
Deficiency	
-Muscle weakness	-Respiratory failure
-Cardiac arrhythmia	
Toxicity	
N/A	
Good sources	
-Fruits (orange juice, bananas, dried fruit)	-Fish
-Yogurt	-Poultry
-Potatoes	-Soy
-Beef, pork	-Vegetables

Table 46: Adapted from: Food and Agriculture Organization and Food and Nutrition Service

Selenium	
Functions	
-Antioxidant	-Regulates thyroid hormone
Deficiency	
-Muscle tenderness	-Pancreas degeneration
-Fragile red blood cells	
Toxicity	
-Weakness	-Liver damage
-Hair and nail loss	
Good sources	
-Whole grains	-Beef, chicken
-Fortified or enriched grains	-Seafood
-Onions	

Table 47: Adapted from: Food and Agriculture Organization and Food and Nutrition Service

Sodium	
*Most Americans are getting too much sodium in their diets through table salt and foods such as breads, pizza, soup and sandwich meat. [66]	
Functions	
-Regulation of fluid and blood volume	-Regulates blood pressure
-Acid-base balance	-Helps with nerve impulse transmission, muscle contraction and heart function
Deficiency	
-Nausea	-Exhaustion
-Cramps	-Possible respiratory failure
-Apathy	
Toxicity	
-High blood pressure for some	
Good sources	
-Table salt	-Most foods except fruit

Table 48: Adapted from: Food and Agriculture Organization and Food and Nutrition Service

Sulfur	
Functions	
-Essential part of amino acids, thiamine, insulin and biotin -Strong and healthy nails and hair	-Elasticity in the skin
Deficiency	
N/A	
Toxicity	
N/A	
Good sources	
N/A	

Table 49: Adapted from: Food and Agriculture Organization and Food and Nutrition Service

Zinc	
Functions	
-Helps form protein -Needed for growth and development	-Important for immune system, nerve function, blood clotting and reproduction -Digestion and metabolism
Deficiency	
-Decreased wound healing -Hair loss	-Diarrhea -Growth failure
Toxicity	
-Stomach upset -Vomiting	-Dizziness
Good sources	
-Oysters -Beef, pork -Liver -Egg yolk -Seafood	-Whole grains -Fortified or enriched grains -Legumes

Table 50: Adapted from: Food and Agriculture Organization and Food and Nutrition Service

Crossword Puzzle

1) Calcium is necessary for strong _____ and teeth.

2) _____ works with potassium, calcium, and magnesium to help regulate blood pressure.

3) Most people are not getting enough _____ in their diets.

4) Potassium helps with acid-base balance and _____ contractions.

5) A good source of _____ is table salt.

6) ____ transports oxygen throughout the body for energy production.

7) A deficiency of _____ can cause goiter, which is an enlargement of the thyroid gland in the neck.

8) Selenium acts as an _____ which can help prevent cancer.

9) Non-heme (non-blood) iron is found in _____ products.

10) Heme (blood) iron is found in _____ products.

11) Bananas and orange juice are good sources of _____.

12) Good sources of chromium, copper, non-heme iron, magnesium, manganese, phosphorus, selenium and zinc are whole _____.

Matching Game   Draw a line to the appropriate answer.

Heme

1) A deficiency in Calcium can lead to _____, which is a softening and weakening of the bones.

Flouride

2) This mineral helps with glucose metabolism.

Rickets

3) ____ (blood) iron is better absorbed than non-heme iron.

Antioxidants

4) Calcium, chloride, magnesium, phosphorus, potassium, and sodium are _____ that provide an acid-base balance in the body.

Calcium

5) This mineral resists acid and decay for healthy teeth.

Chromium

6) Vegetarians may require an ____ mineral supplement (as well as B12)

Electrolytes

7) Adequate _____ (and vitamin D) can help prevent osteoporosis.

Anemia

8) Selenium and zinc are minerals that act as _____.

Iron

9) A deficiency in iron can lead to _____.

Sodium

10) Most Americans are consuming too much of this mineral.

Key for crossword puzzle:

1) Bones
2) Sodium
3) Calcium
4) Muscle
5) Chloride
6) Iron
7) Iodine
8) Antioxidant
9) Plant
10) Animal
11) Potassium
12) Grains

Key for matching game:

1) Rickets
2) Chromium
3) Heme
4) Electrolytes
5) Flouride
6) Iron
7) Calcium
8) Antioxidants
9) Anemia
10) Sodium

Well, that was fun! I just want to add a few more areas to the micronutrient section to include electrolytes, vegetarian diets and antioxidants.

Electrolytes are certain minerals that have an electrical charge to them. [67] Electrolytes are very important for the body because they help balance the amount of water in the body and acidity levels of blood. They also affect muscle function. Again, minerals have to be obtained from food and drinks and the more fluid you lose through exercise and other activities, the more you will need them.

Electrolytes include calcium, chloride, magnesium, phosphorus, potassium and sodium. [68]

Vegetarians will need to pay close attention to certain vitamins and minerals depending on what animal sources they are excluding. These mainly include Vitamin B12, iron, calcium and Vitamin D.

We're going to talk about antioxidants in detail in our next chapter, but I did want to briefly discuss them here since certain vitamins and minerals act as antioxidants:

Antioxidants are found naturally in foods and can help prevent the formation of free radicals, according to National Institutes of Health (NIH). [69] Free radicals cause cell damage, which can eventually lead to cancer and other health problems. Antioxidants help prevent cell damage/free radical damage, which means they may help prevent cancer and other diseases. [69]

Some vitamins and minerals that act as antioxidants include beta-carotene (a precursor of Vitamin A), Vitamin C and Vitamin E. Neat! [69]

Please don't worry about how vague I am being, we'll talk more in detail in the next chapter.

Drum roll please......   my favorite chapter is coming up! Functional foods!

Chapter 13

Functional Foods

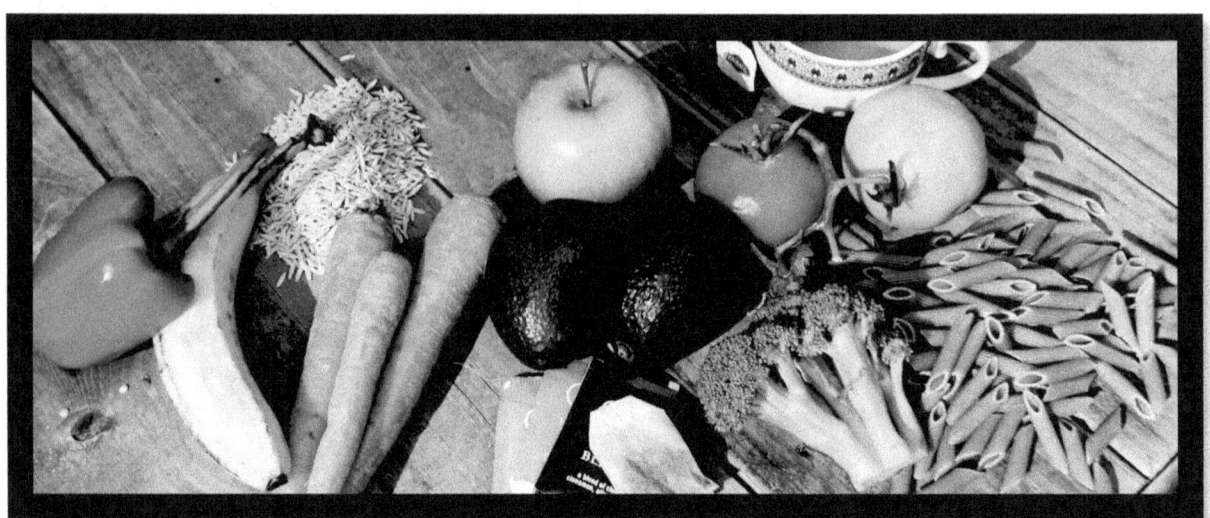

This is my faaaaavorite section! It excites me so and I loooove learning about functional foods and how it can help prevent nutrition-related diseases beyond basic nutrition.

Let's define a few areas first:

<u>Functional food</u>- The Academy of Nutrition and Dietetics defines functional food as "a food that provides additional health benefits that may reduce disease risk and/or promote good health." [70] These can include foods such as bioactive carbohydrates, antioxidants, phytochemicals, dietary fiber, prebiotics, probiotics, starches, functional lipids, functional beverages, vitamins and minerals.

<u>Phytochemical</u>- broad term consisting of plant-derived components that may help protect against disease. These include compounds such as flavonoids, catechins, isoflavones, phenolic acids, flavonols and proanthocyanidins. They are found in foods such as fruits, vegetables, legumes, whole grains, tea and grapes. [71]

<u>Free radical</u>- causes damage to DNA and cells due to oxygen interacting with unpaired electrons on the free radicals, which can lead to cancer, as stated by National Cancer Institute (NCI).[72] Antioxidants help prevent the cell damage caused by free radicals. [72]

<u>Antioxidant</u>- substances found in many fruits and vegetables that help prevent oxidative damage to cells caused by free radicals. These include beta-carotene, lutein, lycopene, selenium, Vitamin A, Vitamin C and Vitamin E. [73]

Functional foods may help prevent our bodies from breaking down prematurely. That's why fruits, vegetables, legumes and whole grains are so important in our diets.

Confession: For the first two-thirds of my college career, I was still only focused on calories. I would eat chips and just count the 200 calories. Then eat other empty calories and count the calories. When I thought about it, I would take a multivitamin/mineral (MVM). Junk food, preservatives, processed foods, etc, etc. But I stayed within my calories, gosh durnit! As the years went by, I noticed I was getting sick more often, feeling run-down easier, etc. All those years of eating junk was breaking my body down prematurely. And that's when I started to learn about functional foods in my classes and I started to TRULY let the nutrition classes sink in. Yes, you lose weight by decreasing your calories and that is important. However, eating 150 calories in junk food instead of 150 calories in healthier options makes a BIG difference in our long-term health, whether you are hitting your calorie goals or not.

Most important is overall health through a variety and balance of beneficial foods such as fruits, vegetables, legumes and whole grains.

And they may help protect against cancer, heart disease and obesity. [74]

And you can't isolate most functional foods; they work together through whole foods.

And if you look closely, you'll likely find something that pertains to you that you might be looking to prevent, such as overweight/obesity! For example, probiotics and insoluble fiber help produce short-chain fatty acids, which have an appetite-suppressant effect on the brain. Another example, medium-chain fatty acids may help in weight loss by breaking down fat through activation of lipase enzyme. And you might find some other fun facts as well!

And

And, And!!

Here are some handy-dandy functional foods, and their potential benefits, to take a gander at:

Category: Capsicum

Capsicum [75]

Potential Benefits:

- Helps prevent free radical damage
- Analgesic (painkiller)

Common Sources: bell peppers, hot peppers

Category: Carotenoids

Beta-carotene (pre-curser of Vitamin A) [74]

Potential Benefits:

- Prevents cell damage from free radicals
- Promotes antioxidant defense

Common Sources: Carrots, pumpkin, sweet potatoes, cantaloupe, dark green leafy vegetables, tomatoes

Lutein [74]

Potential Benefits:

- Eye health

Common Sources: Kale, collards, spinach, corn, eggs, citrus fruits

Lycopene[73,74]

Potential Benefits:

- Helps prevent DNA and cell damage
- May help lower risk of prostate cancer

Common Sources: Tomatoes, processed tomato products, watermelon, red and pink grapefruit

Category: Dietary Fiber

Beta-glucan [75]

(FDA approved health claim)

Potential Benefits:

- May reduce risk of heart disease

Common Sources: Oat bran, oatmeal, barley, rye

Insoluble fiber [74,75]

Potential Benefits:

- Digestive health
- May help reduce cancer
- Feelings of fullness, so reduces food consumption
- Blood glucose management.
- Reduction in appetite, so less calorie intake
- Forms small-chain fatty acids, which has appetite-suppressing effect on the brain

Common Sources: Fruit skins and seeds, whole wheat bread, brown rice, wheat bran

Resistant starches [75]

Potential Benefits:

- Better blood glucose control
- Reduces fat accumulation
- Helps lower blood cholesterol levels

Common Sources: Cooked and cooled foods such as potatoes, rice, tortillas, pasta. Whole grains, seeds and legumes. Under-ripe bananas.

Soluble fiber

(FDA approved health claim)

Potential Benefits:

- May reduce risk of heart disease and certain cancers
- Improves glucose, cholesterol and lipid profiles, so helps prevent against obesity, diabetes, atherosclerosis and cancer

Common Sources: Oatmeal, nuts, peas, beans, apples, citrus fruits, psyllium seed husks

Whole grains

(FDA approved health claim)

Potential Benefits:

- May reduce risk of heart disease and certain cancers.
- Supports healthy blood glucose levels.

Common Sources: Whole grain cereal, whole wheat bread, oatmeal, brown rice

Category: Fatty Acids

Conjugated linoleic acid (CLA) [75]

Potential Benefits:

- Potential maintenance of desirable body composition
- Immune health

Common Sources: Beef and lamb, some cheese

Medium-chain fatty acids [73]

- Potential Benefits:
- Possibly helps reduce body mass index, hip circumference and waist-to-hip ratio
- Helps reduce LDL levels
- Reduces fat accumulation through lipase enzyme

Common Sources: Whole milk, cheese, yogurt

Monounsaturated fatty acids (MUFAs)

(FDA approved health claim) [75]

Potential Benefits:

- May help reduce risk of heart disease
- Reduces total cholesterol and lowered LDL cholesterol levels

Common Sources: Olive oil, canola oil, nuts, avocado

Polyunsaturated fatty acid (PUFAs) / Omega-3 fatty acids: DHA/EPA, ALA

(FDA approved health claim) [75,77]

Potential Benefits:

- Helps lower cholesterol, triglycerides, blood pressure and arthritis
- Appetite- reducing effect
- Supports healthy mental function throughout life
- May help reduce depression, ADHD and aggression
- Heart and eye health
- Required for brain growth and development in infants

Common Sources: Walnuts, salmon, tuna, fish oil, flaxseed, flaxseed oil

Category: Flavonoids

Anthocyanidins [74]

Potential Benefits:

- Antioxidant defense against free radicals
- Supports healthy brain function

Common Sources: Berries, red grapes, cherries

Flavonols- Catechins [73,74]

Potential Benefits:

- Heart health
- Antibacterial
- Decreases risk of cancer, inflammation and atherosclerosis

Common Sources: Tea, dark chocolate, grapes, cocoa, apples, vinegar

Flavonols- Quercetin [74]

Potential Benefits:

- Helps prevent free radical damage and helps with antioxidant defense, so lowered cancer risk

Common Sources: Onions, garlic, apples, tea, broccoli

Flavanones [74]

Potential Benefits:

- Helps prevent free radical damage and helps with antioxidant defense, so lowered cancer risk

Common Sources: Citrus fruits

Proanthocyanidins

Potential Benefits:

- Heart and urinary tract health

Common Sources: Cranberries, cocoa, apples, strawberries, red and purple grapes, peanuts, cinnamon, tea, dark chocolate

Resveratrol [75]

Potential Benefits:

- Slows LDL oxidation and reduced cancer risk

Common Sources: Red and purple grapes, peanuts.

Category: Phytoestrogens

Isoflavones [75]

Potential Benefits:

- Bone, immune and brain health
- Decreases menopause effects with estradiol structure without negative side effects of estradiol (estrogen)
- Decreases LDL, increases HDL and antioxidant effect, so reduced risk of cancer

Common Sources: Soybeans, soy based foods

Lignans[75]

Potential Benefits:

- Heart and immune health

Common Sources: Flaxseeds, rye, seeds, nuts, broccoli, cauliflower, carrots

Category: Plant Stanols and Sterols

Stanols and sterols (FDA approved health claim) [75]

Potential Benefits:

- May help reduce risk of heart disease

Common Sources: Corn, soybeans, wheat, fortified foods and drinks

Category: Prebiotics - food for the intestinal bacteria

Inulin and oligosaccharides [75]

Potential Benefits:

Healthy digestive health and growth of beneficial bacteria in gut.

- Reduces risk of cancer, heart disease, obesity and diabetes
- Helps with calcium absorption

Common Sources: Whole grains, onions, garlic, some fruits, honey, bananas, artichoke, fortified foods and drinks

Category: Probiotics- the actual bacteria that is found in foods and raises intestinal bacteria counts in a beneficial way.

Lactobacilli and bifidobacterium [75]

Potential Benefits:

- Promotes immunity through IgA and natural killer cells
- Produces short-chain fatty acids which has appetite- suppressant effects on brain
- Helps reduce risk of cancer
- Produces anti-microbials
- Digestive health

Common Sources: Certain yogurts and other cultured products, yeast

Category: Soy Protein

Soy protein [73]

(FDA approved health claim)

Potential Benefits:

- May help reduce risk of heart disease
- Reduces cholesterol by binding bile for secretion
- Partial replacement of soy with animal helps decrease cholesterol and saturated fats

Common Sources: Soybeans and soy based products

Category: Sulfides and Thiols

Diallyl sulfide and allyl methyl trisulfide [74]

Potential Benefits:

- May help detoxify unhealthy compounds
- May help heart and immunity

Common Sources: Garlic, onions, leeks, scallions

Dithiolethiones[74]

Potential Benefits:

- May contribute to healthy immunity

Common Sources: Cruciferous vegetables: broccoli, cabbage, bok choy, collards

Sulforaphane [74]

Potential Benefits:

- May help detoxify unhealthy compounds
- Supports antioxidant defense

Common Sources: Cauliflower, broccoli, cabbage, kale, horseradish

Category: Vitamins and Minerals [74]

Vitamin A

Potential Benefits:

- Protection of cells from free radicals

Common Sources: Liver, dairy products, fish

Vitamin C

Potential Benefits:

- Protection of cells from free radicals

Common Sources: Bell peppers, citrus fruits

Vitamin E

Potential Benefits:

- Protection of cells from free radicals

Common Sources: Oils, fortified cereals, sunflower seeds, mixed nuts

Selenium

Potential Benefits:

- Helps prevent free radical damage to cells, so reduced cancer risk

Common Sources: Fish, red meat, whole grains, garlic, liver, eggs

Since I threw a lot of information at you, I wanted to include another set of activities!

Go through the tables and help fill in the class of functional food depending on what potential benefits it imparts. I'll provide the answers at the very bottom of the exercise.

Fill-in-the-Blank Game

Answers are at the bottom of the game.

May help reduce the risk of cancer. Tip: Look for any areas that mention antioxidants, preventing cell damage, stopping free radicals, helping reduce the risk of cancer.

1) B _ _ _ - C _ _ _ _ _ _ _ _
    (Found in: Carrots, pumpkin, sweet potatoes, cantaloupe, spinach, tomatoes)

2) L _ _ _ _ _ _ _ _
    (Found in: Tomatoes, processed tomato products, watermelon, red and pink grapefruit)

3) I _ _ _ _ _ _ _ _ _ _   F _ _ _ _ _
    (Found in: Fruit skins and seeds, whole wheat bread, brown rice, wheat bran, corn bran)

4) S _ _ _ _ _ _ _   F _ _ _ _ _
    (Found in: Oatmeal, nuts, peas, beans, apples, citrus fruits, psyllium seed husks)

5) W _ _ _ _ _ G _ _ _ _ _ _
    (Found in: Whole grain cereal, whole wheat bread, oatmeal, brown rice)

6) A _ _ _ _ _ _ _ _ _ _ _ _ _
    (Found in: Berries, red grapes, cherries)

7) F _ _ _ _ _ _ _ _ - Q _ _ _ _ _ _ _ _
    (Found in: Onions, garlic (also antimicrobial 83) , apples, tea, broccoli)

8) F _ _ _ _ _ _ _ _ - C _ _ _ _ _ _ _ _ _
    (Found in: Tea, dark chocolate, grapes, cocoa, apples)

9) F _ _ _ _ _ _ _ _ _
    (Found in: Citrus fruits)

10) R _ _ _ _ _ _ _ _ _ _ _
    (Found in: Red and purple grapes, peanuts)

11) S _ _ _ _ _ _ _ _ _ _ _
    (Found in: Cauliflower, broccoli, cabbage, kale, horseradish)

12) V _ _ _ _ _ _ _ A
  (Found in: liver, dairy products, fish)

13) V _ _ _ _ _ _ _ C
  (Found in: Bell peppers, citrus fruits)

14) V _ _ _ _ _ _ _ E
  (Found in: Oils, fortified cereals, sunflower seeds, mixed nuts)

15) S _ _ _ _ _ _ _ _
  (Found in: Fish, red meat, whole grains, garlic, liver, eggs)

16) C _ _ _ _ _ _ _ _
  (Found in: Bell peppers, hot peppers)

17) I _ _ _ _ _ _ and O _ _ _ _ _ _ _ _ _ _ _ _ _ _ _ _ _
  (Found in:Whole grains, onions, garlic, some fruits, honey, bananas, artichoke, fortified foods/drinks)

18) L _ _ _ _ _ _ _ _ _ _ _ and B _ _ _ _ _ _ _ _ _ _ _ _ _
  (Found in: Certain yogurts and other cultured products)

19) I _ _ _ _ _ _ _ _ _ _ _
  (Found in: Soybeans, soy based foods)

May help prevent heart disease. Tip: Look for any areas that mentions actions such as decreasing atherosclerosis, decreasing LDL, decreasing triglycerides, decreasing blood pressure, increasing HDL, improving fat profiles.

1) B _ _ _ _ - G _ _ _ _ _ _
  (Found in: Oat bran, oatmeal, barley, rye)

2) S _ _ _ _ _ _ _ F _ _ _ _ _
  (Found in: Oatmeal, nuts, peas, beans, apples, citrus fruits, psyllium seed husks)

3) W _ _ _ _ _ G _ _ _ _ _
  (Found in: Whole grain cereal, whole wheat bread, oatmeal, brown rice)

4) R _ _ _ _ _ _ _ _ S _ _ _ _ _ _ _
  (Found in: Potatoes, rice)

5) M _ _ _ _ _ _ _ _ _ _ _ _ _ _ _ _ F _ _ _ _ _ A _ _ _ _ _
    (Found in: Olive oil, canola oil, nuts)

6) P _ _ _ _ _ _ _ _ _ _ _ _ _ _ _ _ F _ _ _ _ _ A _ _ _ _ _ _
    (Found in: Walnuts, salmon, tuna, fish oil, flaxseed, flaxseed oil)

7) M _ _ _ _ _ _ - C _ _ _ _ _ _ F _ _ _ _ _ A _ _ _ _ _
    (Found in: Milk, cheese, yogurt)

8) F _ _ _ _ _ _ _ _ _ - C _ _ _ _ _ _ _ _ _
    (Found in: Tea, dark chocolate, grapes, cocoa, apples)

9) P _ _ _ _ _ _ _ _ _ _ _ _ _ _ _ _ _ _
    (Found in: Cranberries, cocoa, apples, strawberries, red and purple grapes, peanuts, cinnamon, tea, dark chocolate)

10) R _ _ _ _ _ _ _ _ _ _ _
    (Found in: Red and purple grapes, peanuts)

11) D _ _ _ _ _ _ _ _ S _ _ _ _ _ _ _ and A _ _ _ _ _ M _ _ _ _ _ T _ _ _ _ _ _ _ _ _
    (Found in: Garlic, onions, leeks, scallions)

12) S _ _ _ _ _ _ _ _ and S _ _ _ _ _ _ _ _
    (Found in: Corn, soy, wheat, fortified foods/drinks)

13) I _ _ _ _ _ _ _ and O _ _ _ _ _ _ _ _ _ _ _ _ _ _ _ _ _ _ _
    (Found in: Whole grains, onions, garlic, some fruits, honey, bananas, artichoke, fortified foods/ drinks)

14) I _ _ _ _ _ _ _ _ _ _ _
    (Found in: Soybeans, soy based foods)

15) L _ _ _ _ _ _ _
    (Found in: Flaxseeds, rye, seeds, nuts, broccoli, cauliflower, carrots)

16) S _ _ _ P _ _ _ _ _ _ _
    (Found in: Soybeans and soy based products)

May help with weight health. Tip: Look for any areas that mention feelings of fullness, reduced food consumption, reduction in appetite, improved fat profiles.

1) I _ _ _ _ _ _ _ _ _ F _ _ _ _ _
(Found in: Fruit skins and seeds, whole wheat bread, brown rice, wheat bran, corn bran)

2) S _ _ _ _ _ _ _ F _ _ _ _ _
(Found in: Oatmeal, nuts, peas, beans, apples, citrus fruits, psyllium seed husks)

3) W _ _ _ _ _ G _ _ _ _ _ _
(Found in: Whole grain cereal, whole wheat bread, oatmeal, brown rice)

4) R _ _ _ _ _ _ _ _ _ S _ _ _ _ _ _ _
(Found in: Potatoes, rice)

5) P _ _ _ _ _ _ _ _ _ _ _ _ _ _ _ _ F _ _ _ _ _ A _ _ _ _ _
(Found in: Walnuts, salmon, tuna, fish oil, flaxseed, flaxseed oil)

6) C _ _ _ _ _ _ _ _ _ _ L _ _ _ _ _ _ _ _ A _ _ _ _
(Found in: Beef and lamb, some cheese)

7) M _ _ _ _ _ _ - C _ _ _ _ _ F _ _ _ _ _ A _ _ _ _ _
(Found in: Milk, cheese, yogurt)

8) I _ _ _ _ _ _ _ and O _ _ _ _ _ _ _ _ _ _ _ _ _ _ _ _ _
(Found in: Whole grains, onions, garlic, some fruits, honey, bananas, artichoke, fortified foods/drinks)

9) L _ _ _ _ _ _ _ _ _ _ _ and B _ _ _ _ _ _ _ _ _ _ _ _ _ _ _ _
(Found in: Certain yogurts and other cultured products)

May help with digestive health

1) I _ _ _ _ _ _ _ _ _ F _ _ _ _ _
(Found in: Fruit skins and seeds, whole wheat bread, brown rice, wheat bran, corn bran)

2) I _ _ _ _ _ _ and O _ _ _ _ _ _ _ _ _ _ _ _ _ _ _ _ _
    (Found in: Whole grains, onions, garlic, some fruits, honey, bananas, artichoke, fortified foods and drinks)

3.) L _ _ _ _ _ _ _ _ _ _ _ _ and B _ _ _ _ _ _ _ _ _ _ _ _ _ _ _ _ _ _
    (Found in: Certain yogurts and other cultured products)

May help with blood glucose levels

1) I _ _ _ _ _ _ _ _ _ _ _ F _ _ _ _ _
    (Found in: Fruit skins and seeds, whole wheat bread, brown rice, wheat bran, corn bran)

2) S _ _ _ _ _ _ _ F _ _ _ _ _
    (Found in: Oatmeal, nuts, peas, beans, apples, citrus fruits, psyllium seed husks)

3) W _ _ _ _ _ G_ _ _ _ _ _
    (Found in: Whole grain cereal, whole wheat bread, oatmeal, brown rice)

4) R _ _ _ _ _ _ _ _ S _ _ _ _ _ _ _ _
    (Found in: Potatoes, rice)

5) I _ _ _ _ _ _ and O _ _ _ _ _ _ _ _ _ _ _ _ _ _ _ _ _ _
    (Found in: Whole grains, onions, garlic, some fruits, honey, bananas, artichoke, fortified foods/drinks)

May help with increased immunity

1) C _ _ _ _ _ _ _ _ _ _ L _ _ _ _ _ _ _ _ A _ _ _ _
    (Found in: Beef and lamb, some cheese)

2) D _ _ _ _ _ _ _ S _ _ _ _ _ _ _ _ and A _ _ _ _ _ M _ _ _ _ _ T _ _ _ _ _ _ _ _ _
    (Found in: Garlic, onions, leeks, scallions)

3) D _ _ _ _ _ _ _ _ _ _ _ _ _ _ _ _ _ _
    (Found in: Cruciferous vegetables: broccoli, cabbage, bok choy, collards)

4) L _ _ _ _ _ _ _ _ _ _ _ _ and B _ _ _ _ _ _ _ _ _ _ _ _ _ _
     (Found in: Certain yogurts and other cultured products)

5) I _ _ _ _ _ _ _ _ _ _ _
     (Found in: Soy beans, soy based foods)

6) L _ _ _ _ _ _ _
     (Found in: Flaxseeds, rye, seeds, nuts, broccoli, cauliflower, carrots)

May help with mental function

1) P _ _ _ _ _ _ _ _ _ _ _ _ _ _ _ _ F _ _ _ _ _ A _ _ _ _ _
     (Found in: Walnuts, salmon, tuna, fish oil, flaxseed, flaxseed oil)

2) A _ _ _ _ _ _ _ _ _ _ _ _
     (Found in: Berries, red grapes, cherries)

3) I _ _ _ _ _ _ _ _ _ _ _
     (Found in: Soybeans, soy based foods)

May help as an antimicrobial/antibacterial

1) F _ _ _ _ _ _ _ _ _- C _ _ _ _ _ _ _ _ _
     (Found in: Tea, dark chocolate, grapes, cocoa, apples)

2) L _ _ _ _ _ _ _ _ _ _ _ _ and B _ _ _ _ _ _ _ _ _ _ _ _ _ _
     (Found in: Certain yogurts and other cultured products)

May help prevent inflammation/arthritis

1) P _ _ _ _ _ _ _ _ _ _ _ _ _ _ _ _ F _ _ _ _ _ A _ _ _ _ _
     (Found in: Walnuts, salmon, tuna, fish oil, flaxseed, flaxseed oil)

2) F _ _ _ _ _ _ _ _ _- C _ _ _ _ _ _ _ _ _
     (Found in: Tea, dark chocolate, grapes, cocoa, apples)

May help with bone health

1) I _ _ _ _ _ _ and O _ _ _ _ _ _ _ _ _ _ _ _ _ _ _ _
    (Found in: Whole grains, onions, garlic, some fruits, honey, bananas, artichoke, fortified foods/drinks)

2) I _ _ _ _ _ _ _ _ _ _
    (Found in: Soybeans, soy based foods)

May help with urinary tract health

1) P _ _ _ _ _ _ _ _ _ _ _ _ _ _ _ _ _ _
    (Found in: Cranberries, cocoa, apples, strawberries, red and purple grapes, peanuts, cinnamon, tea, dark chocolate)

May help as a natural painkiller

1) C _ _ _ _ _ _ _ _ _
    (Found in: Bell peppers, hot peppers)

May help with eye health

1) L _ _ _ _ _ _
    (Found in: Kale, collards, spinach, corn, eggs, citrus fruits)

2) P _ _ _ _ _ _ _ _ _ _ _ _ _ _ _ _ F _ _ _ _ A _ _ _ _
    (Found in: Walnuts, salmon, tuna, fish oil, flaxseed, flaxseed oil)

Answers for reduced cancer risk: beta-carotene, lycopene, insoluble fiber, soluble fiber, whole grains, anthocyanins, flavonols-quercetin, flavonols- catechin, flavanones, resveratrol, sulforaphane, selenium, Capsicum, inulin and oligosaccharides, isoflavones, isoflavones, Lactobacilli and bifidobacteria

Answers for heart health: beta-glucan, soluble fiber, resistant starches, monounsaturated fatty acids, polyunsaturated fatty acids, medium-chain fatty acids, flavonols-catechins, proanthocyanidins, resveratrol, diallyl sulfide and allyl methyl trisulfide, stanols and sterols, inulin and oligosaccharides, isoflavones, lignans, soy protein

Answers for weight health: insoluble fiber, soluble fiber, whole grains, resistant starches, polyunsaturated fatty acids, conjugated linoleic acid, medium-chain fatty acids, inulin and oligosaccharides, Lactobacilli and bifidobacteria

Answers for digestive health: insoluble fiber, inulin and oligosaccharides, Lactobacilli and bifidobacteria

Answers for blood glucose health: insoluble fiber, soluble fiber, whole grains, resistant starches, inulin and oligosaccharides

Answers for immunity health: conjugated linoleic acid, diallyl sulfide and allyl methyl trisulfide, dithiolthiones, Lactobacilli and bifidobacteria, isoflavones, lignans

Answers for mental function: polyunsaturated fatty acids, anthocyanins, isoflavones

Answers for antimicrobial/antibacterial: flavonols-catechins, Lactobacilli and bifidobacteria

Answers for anti-inflammatory/arthritis: flavonols-catechins, polyunsaturated fatty acids

Answers for bone health: inulin and oligosaccharides, isoflavones

Answers for urinary tract health: proanthocyanidins

Answers for natural painkiller: capsicum

Answers for cavity prevention: sugar alcohols

Answers for eye health: lutein, polyunsaturated fatty acids

Maybe I'm just a nerd, but I just LOVE the functional foods section the best. I don't claim to eat healthy all the time; that's too big of a tall order for me. I do, now, though, try to make more positive choices in life and food, and that's what counts. Small steps towards big goals!

Speaking of all these great foods and health benefits, I think I'm going to whip myself up some salsa really quick to eat as a snack this evening. Seriously, it takes me less than 15 minutes and is packed full of health. I do tend to let it sit in the fridge for at least an hour to let all the flavors meld, but that's up to you.

Here is the recipe. It's classic. It's good. It's packed with health benefits.

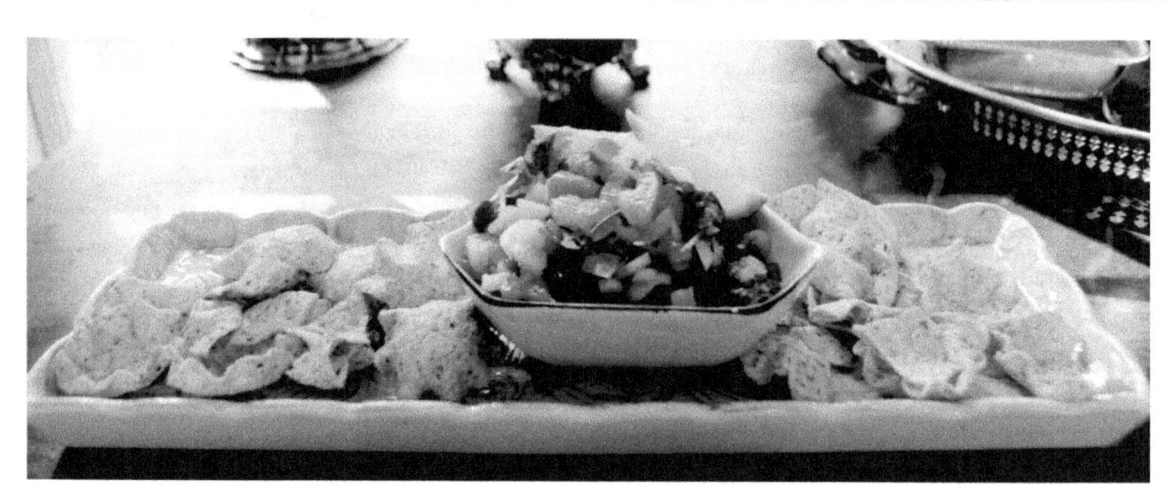

Tomato Salsa

3 large tomatoes

1 small green bell pepper

1 small white onion

3 cloves garlic

1 jalapeno pepper(include some seeds for heat)

1/2 cup fresh cilantro

1 Tbsp lime juice

Salt to taste

Whole grain tortilla chips

1) Chop and combine all ingredients.
2) Refrigerate for about an hour to let the flavors meld.
3) Serve with whole grain tortilla chips.

You can also pulverize the ingredients for a more restaurant style, but I prefer mine chopped, almost like pico de gallo.

Let's see. Potential health benefits include:

- <u>Reduced cancer risk</u> through beta-carotene (tomatoes), lycopene (tomatoes), Vitamin C (bell pepper), selenium (whole grains, garlic), capsicum (bell pepper, hot peppers), inulin/oligosaccharides (garlic) and flavonols-quercetin (garlic, onion).
- <u>Heart health</u> and <u>immunity</u> through diallyl sulfide/allyl methyl trisulfide (garlic, onion) and stanols/sterols (whole grain).
- <u>Digestive health</u> and <u>weight health</u> through inulin/oligosaccharides (garlic, onion, whole grain).

    Nice!!

Mmmm. While I'm on the subject, guacamole also comes to mind, which takes even less time to prepare and is yummy and healthy as well.

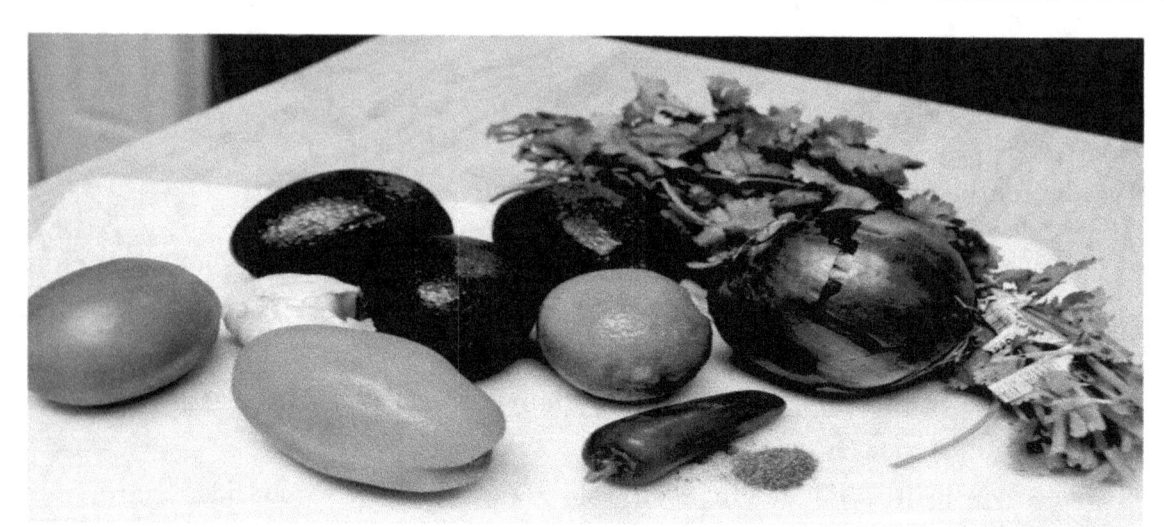

Guacamole

3 avocados, peeled, pitted, mashed

2 roma tomatoes, diced

1 small red onion, diced

3 Tbsp fresh cilantro, chopped

1 garlic clove, minced

1 pinch cayenne pepper

1 lime, juiced

1 tsp salt

Whole grain tortilla chips

1) Mash all of the ingredients together.
2) Refrigerate for at least 1 hour for best flavor.
3) Serve with whole grain tortilla chips.

Potential health benefits include:

- Heart health through monounsaturated fatty acids (avocado).
- Reduced cancer risk through beta-carotene (tomatoes), lycopene (tomatoes), selenium (whole grains, garlic), capsicum (hot peppers) inulin/oligosaccharides (garlic, onion, whole grain) and flavonols-quercetin (garlic, onion).
- Heart health and immunity through diallyl sulfide/allyl methyl trisulfide (garlic, onion) and stanols/sterols (whole grain).
- Digestive health and weight health through inulin/oligosaccharides (garlic, onion, whole grain).

  LOVE!

Let's go ahead and take a look at the potential benefits from the balsamic vinaigrette dressing that we discussed in the chapter on vitamins:

- Heart health through monounsaturated fatty acids (olive oil), flavonols-catechins (vinegar) and diallyl sulfide/allyl methyl trisulfide (garlic).
- Antibacterial effect through flavonols-catechins (vinegar).
- Reduced cancer risk through inulin/oligosaccharides (honey), flavonols-quercetin (garlic), flavonols-catechins (vinegar) and selenium (garlic).
- Digestive health and weight health through inulin/oligosaccharides (honey, garlic).
- Enhanced immunity through diallyl sulfide/allyl methyl trisulfide (garlic).

And, in case you missed this dressing recipe all together, I'll list it here again!

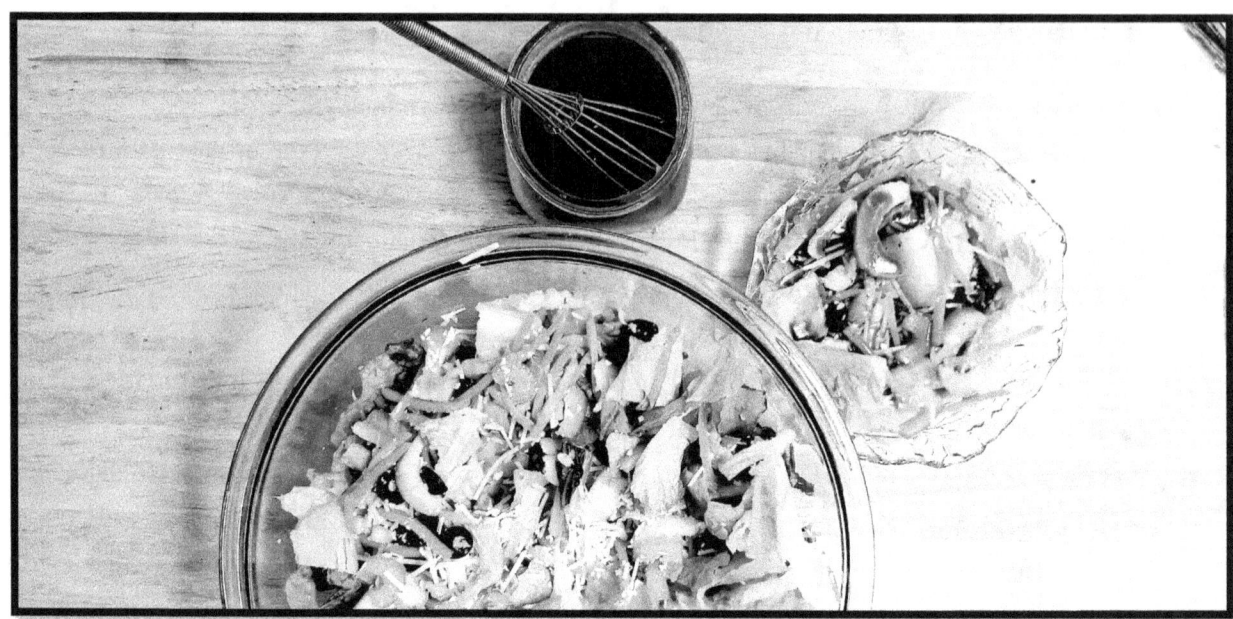

Balsamic Vinaigrette Dressing

2/3 cup olive oil

1/3 cup balsamic vinegar

2 cloves garlic, finely minced

2 Tbsp Dijon mustard (or more to taste)

2 Tbsp honey

½ tsp Worcestershire®

½ tsp hot sauce

¼ tsp salt

¼ tsp pepper

1) Whisk all ingredients together very well.
2) Pour into a mason jar with lid (or any container that has a tight seal).
3) Keep unused dressing in the refrigerator.

Okay, time to move on. Not to worry, though, there is still plenty of interesting stuff to come!

Chapter 14

Potential Contributors to Body Breakdown

As I mentioned in the last chapter, my diet used to be bad, bad, bad. And then my body started prematurely breaking down, down, down. I found a new love in those beautiful functional foods found in whole grains, fruits, vegetables and healthy fats. I am a lover of those whole grains, fruits, vegetables and healthy fats that can help prevent further breakdown and even repair some damage.

Along with my poor food group choices, I ate a ton of processed foods, which helped contribute to my body breakdown. So now I try to find better alternatives. Enough about me from now on, let's just focus on the information and ways we can help YOU and save your body from the same fate!

Note: This chapter contains highly debatable topics. I urge you to please do your own research (choosing from highly reputable sources such as .edu and .gov sites) and come to your own conclusions if you still have concerns.

Overly Processed Foods

According to the Academy of Nutrition and Dietetics (AND), eating an abundance of processed foods can lead to health problems such as high blood pressure, type 2 diabetes and obesity. [78]

Examples of potentially overly processed foods are ready-to-eat foods such as certain deli meats, bacon, packaged snacks, frozen foods and microwaveable dinners.

The problem with overly processed foods is that they tend to contain a high amount of sugar, sodium and fat which can lead to health problems in the long run.

Here are a few tips from AND to keep in mind as you are walking the grocery aisles:

-Look for a better alternative if the first 2-3 ingredients are sugar, maltose, brown sugar, corn syrup, cane sugar, honey or fruit juice concentrate.

-Steer clear of trans fats on the nutrition facts panel and partially hydrogenated vegetable oils in the ingredient list.

-Look for reduced or low sodium, which can reduce sodium content by 40%.

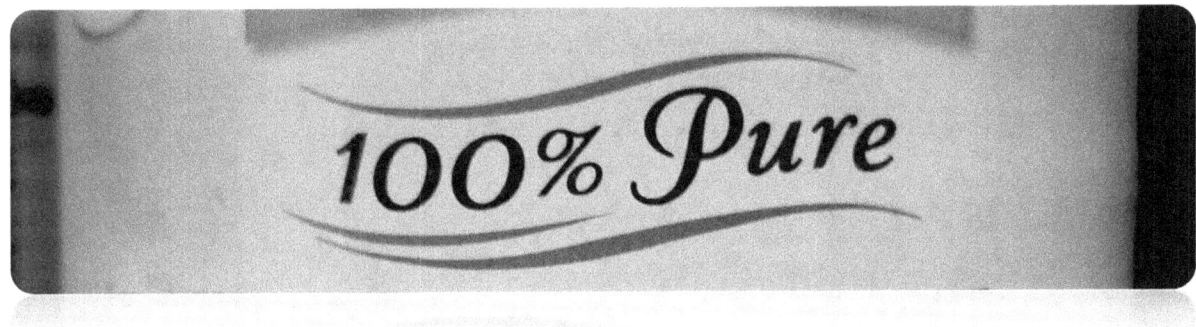

Refined Sugars

Refined sugars come from sugar cane through an extraction process. [79] This is your typical sugar found in foods and drinks such as sodas, cakes, cookies and some cereals. They are high in calories and low in nutritional value, so consuming less of these can help in the prevention of obesity and obesity-related diseases.

Additives: Preservatives

Most processed foods contain additives, such as preservatives. These include foods like snacks, ready-to-eat meals, deli meats and some soups and sauces. [80]

Food additives can help keep food from spoiling prematurely by helping preserve taste, texture and nutrition. They also can help the appearance of foods.

Not all additives are unsafe. Generally Recognized as Safe (GRAS) is a regulation governed by the Food and Drug Administration (FDA) and lists all additives that have been approved by qualified experts and the FDA as safe when used as intended, in small amounts. [81] Key word: small amounts

Some examples of preservatives include: ascorbic acid (Vitamin C- antioxidant), lactic acid, lecithin, sodium citrate, stearic acid, propylene glycol and ascorbyl palmitate (antioxidant).[81]

Your best bet: Search for preservative-free options when available.

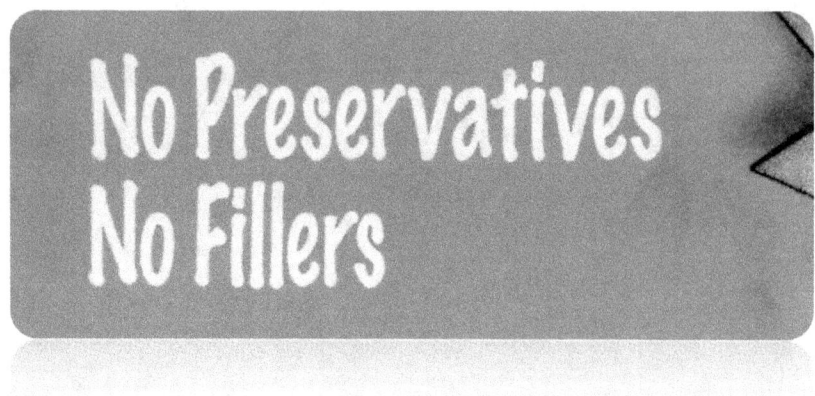

Pesticides

Pesticides are used in order to prevent pests from damaging crops. Some pesticides can cause cancer, nervous system problems and endocrine system problems. [82] However, the US Environmental Protection Agency (EPA) has banned certain pesticides called persistent organic pollutants (POPs) that are known carcinogens. They have also banned other pesticides made with ammonia, chlorine, methanol, arsenic, etc. [82]

Your best bet: If you are concerned about pesticide use, choose United States Department of Agriculture (USDA) organic products since they do not use conventional pesticides or synthetic fertilizers. [83]

Added Hormones and Antibiotics

Hormones and antibiotics have been added to some animal products in order to help the growth rate of the animal.

Hormones: The FDA regulates which hormones are allowed. Hormones are not allowed in poultry or pork, but are allowed in beef. [84] Naturally occurring hormones include estrogen, progesterone and testosterone. The FDA states that these are not added in amounts that would pose harm to humans. [84] Synthetic hormones require testing and only hormones that are found to be at safe levels are allowed.

Antibiotics: The FDA is currently working to voluntarily remove non-medically necessary antibiotics from our food sources due to antimicrobial resistance. [85] Some manufacturers are choosing to remove antibiotics from their meat and poultry and are allowed the label "no antibiotics added."

Your best bet: Again, USDA organic is a great option for some because the meat, poultry, eggs and dairy do not contain antibiotics or growth hormones. [86]

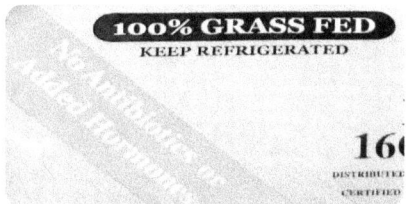
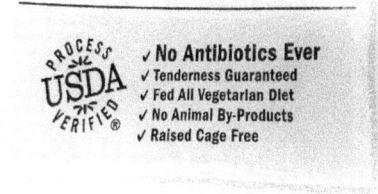

Plastics

Bisphenol A (BPA.) I remember hearing about this word in my elementary organic chemistry class. These are polycarbonate plastics and resins that are used in some water bottles, food storage containers and canned foods. [87] The FDA has found BPA's to be safe at very low levels; however they may have cumulative effects in the body and may have negative health effects on the brain and behavior of infants and children as well as negative effects on blood pressure.[87] The FDA has banned BPA's in baby bottles, sippy cups and packaging for infant formula. It continues to review information and discuss further banning of BPS's with the scientific community. [88]

The National Institutes of Health (NIH) has some recommendations for limiting BPA ingestion: Do not heat up plastic containers in the microwave. Stay away from certain recycled plastics that have a code 3 or 7 on the bottom. Reduce your use of canned foods.

Opt for glass, porcelain or stainless steel containers. Look for containers that say "BPA free." [89]

We'll discuss another set of hot topics next: GMOs and sweeteners.

Chapter 15

Genetically Engineered Foods and Sweeteners

Note: This chapter contains highly debatable topics. I urge you to please do your own research (choosing from highly reputable sources such as .edu and .gov sites) and come to your own conclusions if you still have concerns.

Genetically Engineered Foods (GE)

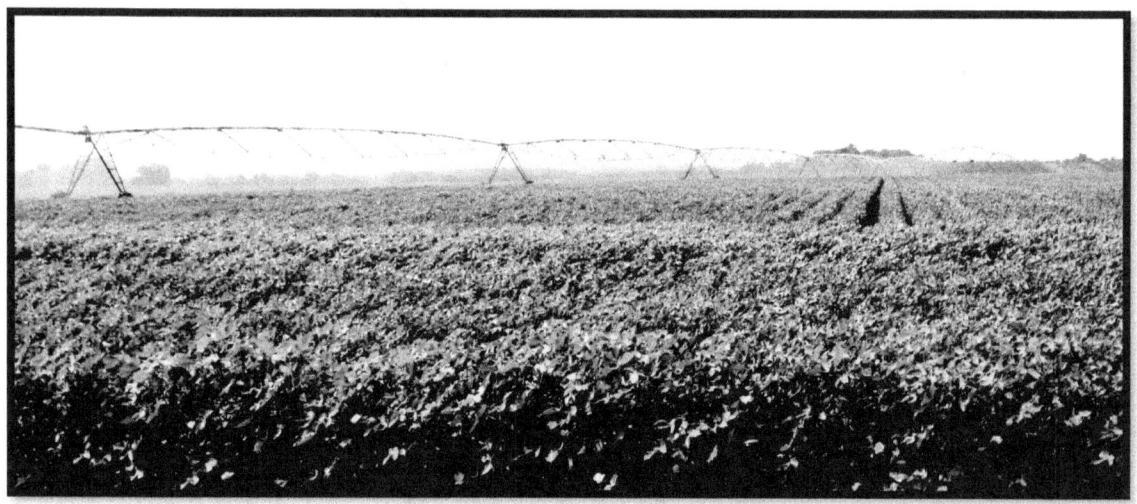

GE foods are created through biotechnology in order to promote enhanced traits in crops. So far there are 10 crops currently available on the market in the United States that may be genetically modified and they include corn (maize), soybeans, cotton, alfalfa, sugar beets, papaya, squash, potato, apple and canola. [90]

2 types of GE crops are herbicide-resistant and insect-resistant. The National Academy of Sciences (NAS) states that herbicide-resistant crops have no substantial adverse effects on animals, soil or water. They also state that insect-resistant crops are harmless to animals and humans. [91]

Due to continued skepticism, however, the NAS recently underwent an updated study on the safety of genetically engineered crops, which was completed May 2016. [91,92] They still found no evidence of any health risks from genetically engineered foods and you can read more about the research methods and conclusions in their free PDF version here:

http://nas-sites.org/ge-crops/

Sweeteners

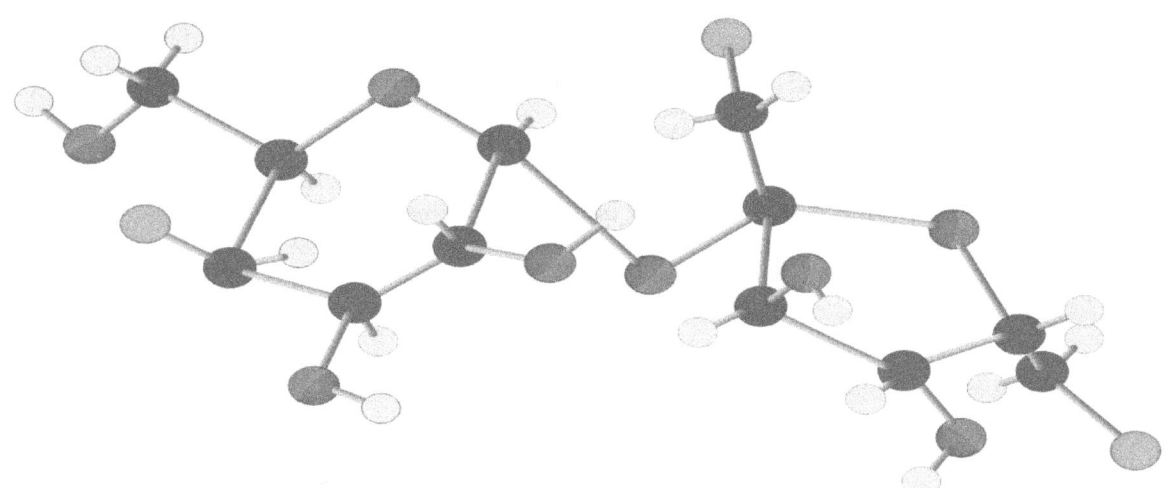

Nonnutritive sweetener- Sucralose

The position statement of the Academy of Nutrition and Dietetics (AND) states that certain nutritive and nonnutritive sweeteners are safe for human consumption when consumed in moderate amounts consistent with a healthy eating plan. [93] This position is also backed up by the American Diabetes Association and National Cancer Institute (NCI).

Nutritive sweeteners contain carbohydrates and calories. They are usually in the form of added sugars and are found in soda, desserts and candy and have greatly added to the obesity epidemic in the United States. [93]

Nonnutritive sweeteners provide 200 to 13,000 times the sweetness of sugar with little to no carbohydrate or calories. [94]

A few of the non-nutritive sweeteners that are FDA approved include saccharin (Sweet'N Low®), aspartame (Equal®), Sucralose (Splenda®), neotame and highly refined stevia. [95] The FDA has established Acceptable Daily Intake (ADI) levels for these sweeteners and it has been found that Americans are well below the ADI level.

Saccharin (Sweet'N Low®)

Saccharin was initially under fire when it was linked to bladder cancer in laboratory rats in the 1970's and a warning label was required on all saccharin products. However, over 30 studies have since found that the mechanism that caused the cancer in rats does not exist in humans. Subsequent human studies have found no clear evidence that saccharin causes cancer in humans, as reported by the NCI. [96] Since 2000, the saccharin warning label has been repealed and a warning label is no longer required. [93]

Aspartame (Equal®)

Aspartame has had over 100 studies performed on its safety and it was concluded that it is safe for human consumption. [96] In 1996, there were some questions between a link between aspartame consumption and brain tumors when aspartame was originally allowed in the United States. However, according to NCI, it was found that the rise in brain tumors was 8 years prior to the approval of aspartame. [96]

Aspartame does contain the amino acid phenylalanine, so if you are phenylalanine sensitive or have phenylketonuria (PKU), then please avoid aspartame. [95]

Sucralose (Splenda®)

With over 100 safety studies, Sucralose was approved by the FDA and there is no evidence of causing harm or cancer to humans. [95]

Stevia

Stveia is plant-based from the leaves of Bertoni, which is found in South America. It has not yet been approved by the FDA in its whole leaf or crude extract form. However, a highly refined stevia form has been approved. [95]

Neotame

Neotame is 7,000 to 13,000 times sweeter than sugar and is approved for use in food. [93] Up-and-coming food and science research is looking into its ability to replace added sugars completely.

Note: Research is ongoing for a better understanding into the potentially positive and/or negative impacts of nonnutritive sweeteners on weight.

Chapter 16

Hormones and Pharmacotherapy

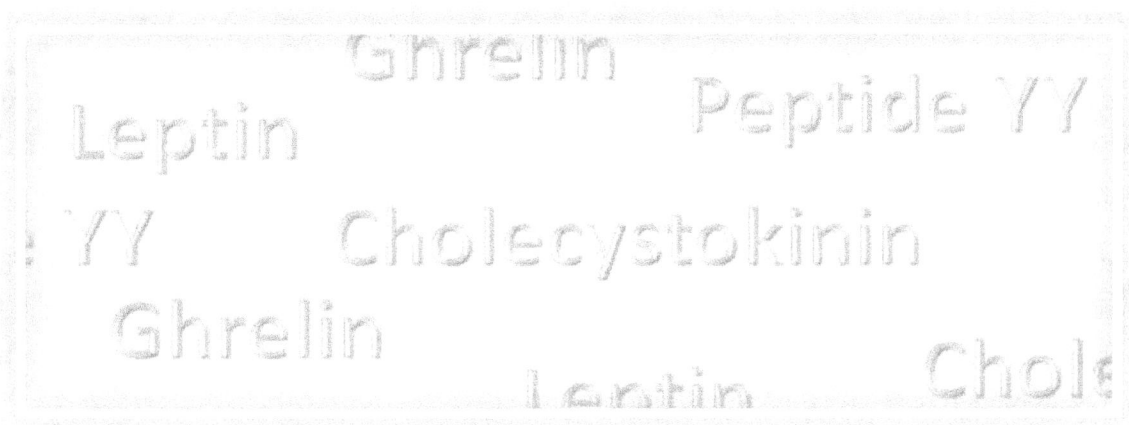

This is a fascinating section; I really like this section.

I've mentioned hormones and hormonal imbalances a few times throughout the book, so I'd like to go ahead and talk about the specifics a little.

There are a few hormones that regulate appetite and satiety. These include hormones such as leptin, ghrelin, cholecystokinin and peptide YY. If a person gains excessive weight, is consistently sleep deprived or deprives themselves of necessary calories through dieting, their hormones tend to become more out of balance, which can lead to further weight gain.

Prevention of excessive weight and obesity is key, but it is not too late for those that are struggling. You can slowly re-set your system one step at a time as mentioned in the nutrition counseling and other sections.

Ghrelin

Ghrelin is known as the "hunger hormone" because it increases hunger and prompts food intake. [97] It is produced in the stomach and affects the hypothalamus (the main regulator of temperature, thirst, hunger, sleep, circadian rhythm, moods, sex drive and other hormones). [97]

Cauter, et al. found that those who do not get enough sleep tend to produce more levels of ghrelin, which can lead to eventual weight gain. [98]

Cholecystokinin

Cholecystokinin is a hormone that is stimulated from the stomach during meals. According to The American Journal of Clinical Nutrition (AJCN), it signals satiation which helps notify the person to stop eating. [99]

When a person tries to go all out and "diet," exclude entire food groups, or starve/ food deprive themselves, they throw off the balance of hormones, such as cholecystokinin. This can lead to even further feelings of hunger, and even more food is needed in order to feel satiated, which leads to further weight gain. [99]

Leptin

Leptin is produced by fat tissue and regulates long-term energy balance. It suppresses the appetite and causes increased energy expenditure. [100]

A review by Klok, et al. reported that obese persons tend to be leptin-resistant, which means that their appetite-suppression capabilities are limited. This can lead to eating more often than they normally would or even may want to eat. [100]

Leptin also is lowered in those with sleep deprivation, which also contributes to weight gain. [98]

Peptide YY

Peptide YY is produced in the stomach and, akin to leptin, it also helps decrease the appetite, which can lead to reduced food intake. [101]

According to The Journal of Physiology (JP), those with low peptide YY levels are more predisposed to the development of obesity. [101]

Peptide YY has been given intravenously and has shown promising results for regulating food intake and reducing appetite. There is also research being conducted on its potential role on increasing energy expenditure. [101]

Our bodies are pretty darn amazing, right? The homeostatic balance that our bodies naturally create is really neat. But if we have thrown off our own homeostatic balance, we have the potential to help lower our weight and lower our health risks one food behavior goal at a time!

What about prescription weight loss meds?

Currently, pharmacotherapy is approved for those with a BMI over 30 (obese) OR with a BMI over 27 (overweight) along with at least one weight-related health problem such as diabetes, high cholesterol or high blood pressure. [102]

A few of the medications include phentermine, lorcaserin and orlistat. [102]

-Phentermine is FDA approved for reducing appetite.

-Lorcaserin is FDA approved and helps with feelings of fullness which leads to reduced food intake.

-Orlistat is FDA approved and inhibits fat absorption up to 30%.

Orlistat also comes in a nonprescription form as well (Alli®) and is FDA approved. Always talk to your doctor before taking any medications, whether over-the-counter or not. [103]

Each of these has potential side effects, so you'll want to discuss your eligibility, types of medications and potential side effects with your doctor.

Please don't read this and just think that pills are the magic answer to your weight. Any person looking to take medications to help them along will still need nutrition counseling to help establish healthy food behaviors. This is essential in order to help keep the weight off after the medication is reduced and eventually stopped. Healthy eating habits and exercise are key in helping to lose weight and keep it off long-term, so please take time to form healthy habits that will last a lifetime.

We've discussed healthy eating habits throughout the book. Now that I'm bringing up exercise, let's go ahead and talk about that. Exercise seems to have a polarizing effect for some. There's no need, I promise. I'm not asking you to go crazy and exercise for 1 hour per day 5 days per week. I'm talking, let's take it slow. Let's go for a walk as a family after dinner 3 nights a week kind of thing. Let's build on our health and fitness goals over time kind of thing.

Chapter 17

Exercise

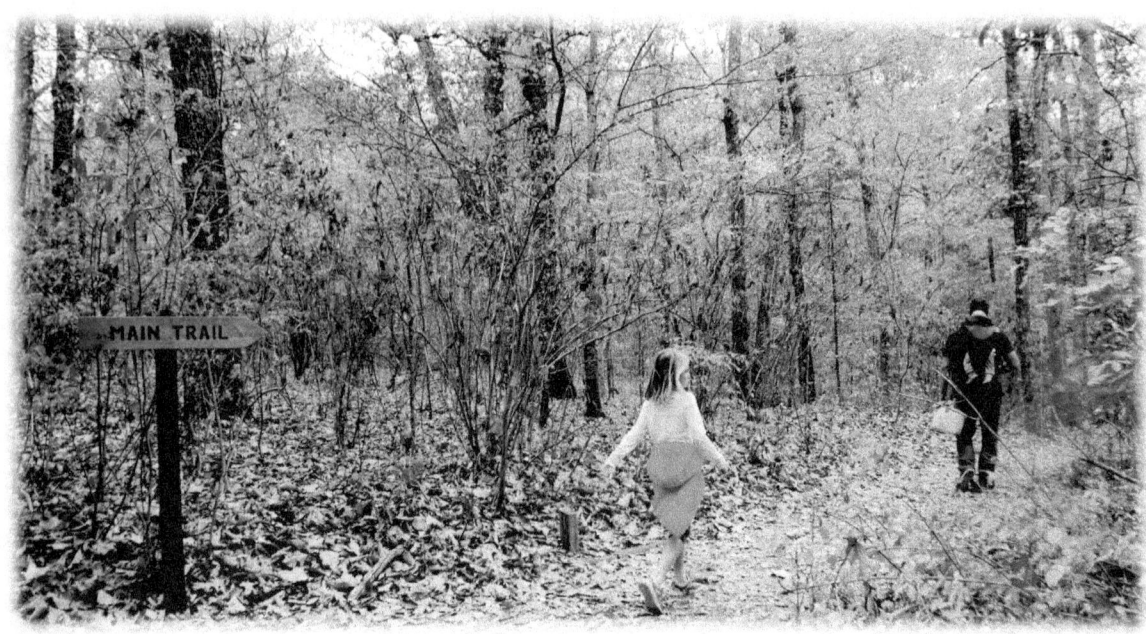

Let me start out by saying that you can gain health benefits from moderate-intensity exercise (brisk walking for example) 60 minutes per week, according to the National Institutes of Health (NIH).[101] That's 2-3 brisk walks, such as keeping up with the kids' leisure bicycling, after dinner with the family. That's not so overwhelming, right? You can do that. I know you can.

The US Department of Health and Human Services (HHS) recommends 2 ½ hours of moderate-intensity exercise (brisk walking) per week or 1 hour 15 minutes of vigorous-intensity exercise per week. Muscle strengthening activities should be included 2 days per week. [104]

However, going from 0 to 100 with nutrition or exercise tends to lead to giving up and feeling even worse about yourself. So do yourself a favor and start slloooowwww. And ALWAYS talk to your doctor before starting any exercise regime.

Use your goal setting technique of small, realistic, achievable goals. Then slowly work up from there. Short bursts of exercise are also beneficial for the body and can add up to total exercise.

Take the stairs instead of the elevator. Go for a walk after dinner a few nights a week. Get out on the playground with your children instead of sitting on the bench. Walk around the parking lot (safely) while your child is at soccer.

Some job sites are even promoting worksite wellness and incorporating physical activity and rewards. Maybe you can check into that or get one started at your job site?

What are some ways you can think to slowly and realistically add a little exercise to your life?

_____

_____

_____

The reasons why exercise is so important are bountiful. Cengage Learning has listed some great benefits:

Potential Benefits of Regular Physical Activity: [105]

1. Reduces premature death from chronic diseases.
2. Reduces risk of heart disease and strengthens heart and lungs.
3. Reduces risk of diabetes.
4. Helps maintain healthy bones with resistance activities such as hiking, dancing and sports.
5. Improves mood, self-image and energy levels.
6. Improves sleep.
7. Improves productivity.
8. Helps with weight control or maintenance.

Keep this in mind as well: Nutrition is very important for weight loss, but exercise is more important when keeping the weight off. The Centers for Disease Control (CDC) reports that those who engage in 60-90 minutes of moderate-intensity exercise per week, while not overeating, tend to keep the weight off. [106]

If you find yourself plateauing (working hard, but the weight still isn't coming off), try mixing up your workouts. Our bodies tend to get used to a routine and will learn to burn less calories doing the same exercise that once helped you burn calories.

Circuit training also helps re-boot the body and really provides a great workout. It uses both weight resistance and physical activity in the same workout. I find that most gyms are set up for circuit training.

You can try about 10-20 repetitions on an exercise machine, then do a short cardio activity for 30-60 seconds, such as jumping jacks, jump rope or jumping in place. Then go on to the next exercise machine and do another 15-20 repetitions, then another cardio activity for 30-60 seconds. Repeat down the line. [107]

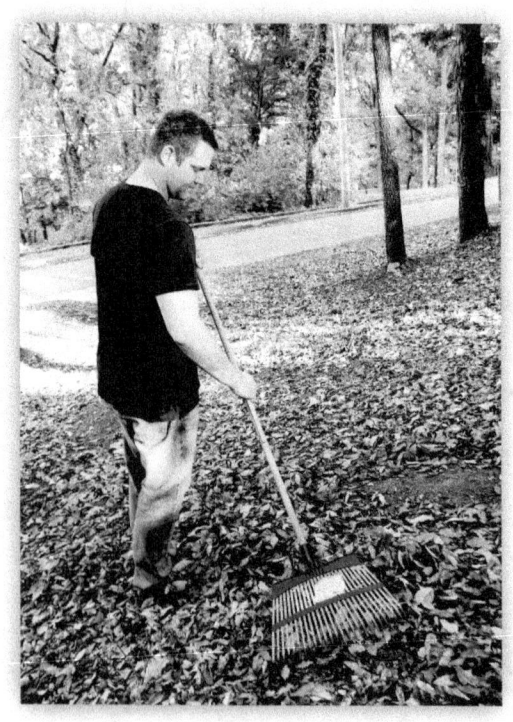

But let's get back to starting slowly and adding any exercise to your life. Earlier you made a list of potential options for adding a little exercise to your life. Below are a few more examples for you. I only added the calories burned for those that find it interesting. I am not requiring any calorie or calories burned counting at all. We're just talking about getting up and moving. [108]

Calories Burned

I got this great list from Harvard Health. Note: The majority of these are categorized as "moderate effort" and "general play" and are based on calories burned when exercising for 30 minutes.

Activity	Clories burned: 125-pound person	Calories burned: 155-pound person	Calories burned: 185-pound person
Aerobics, water	120	149	178
Aerobics, low impact	165	205	244
Aerobics, high impact	210	260	311
Basketball	240	298	355
Bicycling: 12-13.9 mph	240	298	355
Bicycling, Stationary, moderate	210	260	311
Bowling	90	112	133
Circuit Training	240	298	355
Chopping and splitting wood	180	223	266
Dancing, slow	90	112	133
Dancing: moderate	165	205	244
Elliptical Trainer	270	335	400
Frisbee	90	112	133
Gardening	135	167	200
Heavy Cleaning, wash car, windows	135	167	200
Horseback Riding	120	149	178
Ice Skating	210	260	311

Martial Arts	300	372	444
Mowing Lawn, push, power	135	167	200
Playing with kids, moderate effort	120	149	178
Racquetball	210	260	311
Raking Lawn	120	149	178
Rollerblading	210	260	311
Rock Climbing, rappelling	240	298	355
Rope Jumping	300	372	444
Running: 5 mph (12 min/mile)	240	298	355
Running: 10 mph (6 min/mile)	495	614	733
Shoveling Snow, by hand	180	223	266
Soccer	210	260	311
Softball	150	186	222
Swimming	180	223	266
Tai Chi	120	149	178
Tennis	210	260	311
Walking: 4 mph (15 min/mi)	135	167	200
Walk/Jog: jog <10 min.	180	223	266
Weight Lifting	90	112	133
Volleyball	90	112	133

Table 63: Adapted from: Harvard Health Publications

Target Heart Rate and Maximum Heart Rate

Also, for those that care, here is the target heart rate calculation. This can help determine if you are doing too much, and thus straining yourself, or doing too little during exercise.

1. Aim for the lower set of numbers to begin with.
2. These are general guidelines and are based on averages.

I will also provide the maximum heart rate calculation as well, just in case you wanted it.

Age, in years	Target HR Zone (50-85%) Beats per minute (bpm)	Maximum heart rate (100%) Beats per minute (bpm)
20	100-170	200
30	95-162	190
40	90-153	180
50	85-145	170
60	80-136	160
70	75-128	150

Table 64: Adapted from: American Heart Association

Maximum Heart Rate Calculation [109]

220 – age = maximum heart rate

For example: A 50 year old male

220 – 50 = 170 bpm, maximum heart rate

Body Fat Percentage

Your local fitness center may use a tool to measure body fat percentage to help gauge your fitness level. Just keep in mind that some measurement tools can have high error rates, so your best bet is the skin-fold measurement or bioelectrical impedance analysis.

	Women	Men
Essential for life	10-13%	2-5%
Athletes	14-20%	6-13%
Fitness	21-24%	14-17%
Acceptable	25-31%	18-25%
Obese	32+%	26+ %

Table 65: Adapted from: ACE Fitness

Alrighty, let's wrap it up with some follow-up nutrition counseling!

Chapter 18

Follow-up Counseling

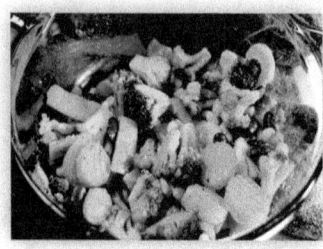 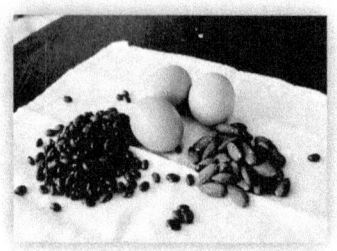 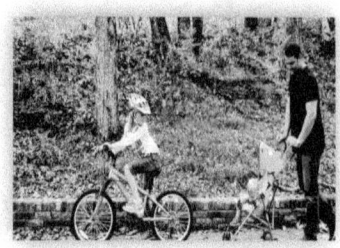

By this point, you hopefully have been working on a nutrition-related goal. Or maybe you are now in the maintenance phase of that goal and have started to work on a new goal. Either way, I want to check in with you!

How did you do on your goal? How do you feel about it?

If you are in the maintenance phase and have started a new goal, then congratulations! You're one step closer to better health and weight goals. If you found that you have struggled, IT IS OKAY. You are okay. Maybe you were trying to take on too much too soon and need to choose a new goal that is more attainable for your current situation.

Let's take a minute to re-assess. Think about everything you had to eat and drink from the time you woke up yesterday to the time you went to bed. Please fill out this table as you think through your day yesterday.

Time	Location	Food or Drink Consumed	Food Group (If not a food group, then write in what it was such as "empty calories")	Serving Size	Feelings at the time; Reason for Eating

Are you finding that you're naturally making better choices? If so, then great! If not, then that is okay, we are all a work in progress. Allow yourself to be human. Recognize that it's okay to make mistakes. Forgive yourself. Just know that you are on your way to making better choices in the future and making a great goal to work toward.

Please go back to your list of food, exercise and lifestyle changes that you would like to make (from Chapter 4) and list them again here. If you have any new changes you would like to make, please list those as well

_____	_____	_____
_____	_____	_____
_____	_____	_____
_____	_____	_____
_____	_____	_____

Choose 1 or 2 that you think are most realistic and attainable for your current situation:

- _____

- _____

Readiness to Change

Test your readininess to change using the ruler and outcomes.

1	2	3	4	5	6	7	8	9	10	11	12

1= not ready

12= ready and motivated

If you find that you're lower on the ruler scale, then please take the time to work through the section of Chapter 4 (just below the ruler) that discusses ways to move forward. If you are ready and motivated, then we're ready to make a new goal!

Remember to narrow down your broad goal using the SMART rules that we discussed earlier:

SMART Rules for Goal Setting:
<ul><li>Specific</li><li>Measurable</li><li>Action-oriented</li><li>Realistic</li><li>Time frame</li></ul>

As always, WRITE YOUR GOAL DOWN, draw boxes to mark off each day, and place it somewhere front and center as a daily reminder.

_____

Let's take a moment to remind ourselves of why we are making changes. [110]

What are some consequences of not making a change in your life?

_____

_____

_____

What are some benefits of making changes? Maybe you will feel better about yourself through a sense of accomplishment. Maybe making positive changes will allow you to have more energy to play with your children or grandchildren.

_____

_____

_____

What are some barriers to making changes? Is there anything standing in your way to one of your goals?

_____

_____

_____

What are some ways to overcome these barriers?

_____

_____

_____

Self-efficacy. I just love that word. The American Psychological Association (APA) states that <u>self-efficacy</u> is the belief you have in yourself in order to follow through to success. [111] What are some skills that you have that can help you succeed?

_____

_____

_____

I'll leave it up to you whether you want to utilize a weight scale on your journey. Some people find it discouraging and others find it encouraging. I will say this, though, that a Cornell University study showed that weighing yourself daily and writing the weight down led to more weight loss, both short- and long-term. [112] Akin to your written goals that you check off each day, you are being more conscious of your choices and holding yourself accountable. This tends to influence our life in positive ways.

Moderation, Balance, Variety

A few final refreshers and tips about moderation, balance and variety (we all knew I wouldn't let us end without mentioning moderation again, right?) :

- Allow yourself time to change your habits. Slowly build on each goal until you have a wealth of healthy food and lifestye choices. This provides slow and consistant weight loss and raises your chances of actually keeping the weight off in the long run.
- Eat until you are satiated (full), not stuffed. It won't be the last time you eat that food item. There will be other days.
- All foods can fit. Just make sure that whole grains, vegetables, fruits, lean proteins and dairy are more predominant in your life in order to help improve your health in both the short and long run.
- Mix up the colors on your dinner plate. Think a variety of colors such as dark green, orange, etc.
- Downsize your plate, bowl and utensil size. When we have huge bowls and plates, we tend to naturally want to fill it up, which can lead to consistant over eating and eventual weight gain.
- Sit down together as a family to eat. This helps to strengthen the family. It also encourages healthier food choices and helps make you more conscious of what and how much you are eating.
- Savor your food. Eat slowly. It leads to feelings of satisfaction and helps you eat less.
- Allow yourself some of life's little pleasures. Sit outside and watch the birds chirp away as you de-stress and soak up the sun. When you are in a better state of mind,

you may find that you choose healthier options and eat less overall, which can help lead to weight loss . [113]

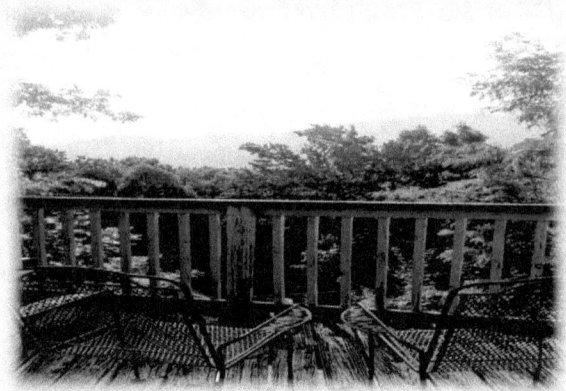

- Think positive thoughts. Praise yourself for all of your positive attributes and recognize that none of us are perfect; we are just looking for progress.
- And lastly, try and find social support through family and friends. Supportive, and even involved, friends and family can have a positive impact to your success in weight and nutrition goals. [114]

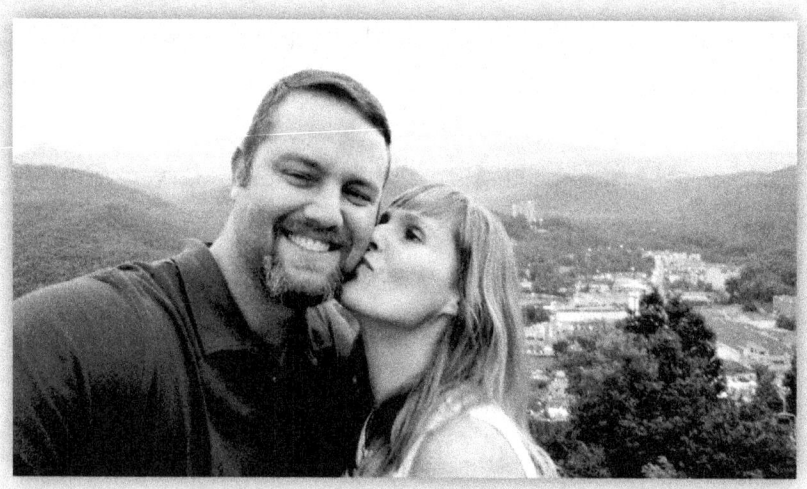

Okay, I think I'm rambling; I'll go ahead and stop now, haha.

I wish you the BEST of luck on your journey to all of your health, weight and fitness goals! I KNOW you can do it; I believe in you!!!

We hope you enjoyed reading this book. For updates on current projects or to follow the author's weekly nutrition blogs, please check out:

shannondeshazer.wordpress.com

Appendix

Acronyms

AMDR- Acceptable Macronutrient Distribution Range

BMI- Body Mass Index

BPA- bisphenol A

CLA- conjugated linoleic acid

DHA- docosahexaenoic acid

DNA- deoxyribonucleic acid

EPA- eicosapentaenoic acid

FDA- U.S. Food and Drug Administration

GE- genetically engineered

GMO- genetically modified organisms

GRAS- Generally Recognized as Safe

HDL- high-density lipoprotein

HHS- Health and Human Services

LDL- low-density lipoprotein

MUFA- monounsaturated fatty acid

PUFA- polyunsaturated fatty acid

RNA- ribonucleic acid

SMART- specific, measurable, action-oriented, realistic, time frame

TSH- thyroid stimulating hormone

USDA- U.S. Department of Agriculture

Glossary

<u>Additives</u>- substances added to foods to prevent spoiling and improve appearance of foods.

<u>Allyl methyl trisulfide</u>- acts as an antioxidant to help detoxify unhealthy compounds.

<u>Amino acids</u>- building blocks of protein.

<u>Analgesic</u>- painkiller.

<u>Anemia</u>- lack of enough healthy blood cells to carry oxygen throughout the body.

<u>Anthocyanin</u>- acts as an antioxidant to protect against free radicals.

<u>Antibiotics</u>- substances used to fight bacterial infections.

<u>Antioxidant</u>- can help prevent the destruction of cells caused by free radicals.

<u>Ascorbic acid</u>- Vitamin C; water soluble vitamin to promote collagen synthesis and wound healing and acts as an antioxidant for potential protection of cells from free radicals.

<u>Aspartame</u>- Equal®; a nonnutritive sweetener that contains phenylalanine.

<u>Atherosclerosis</u>- fatty plaque buildup in the arteries.

<u>Beta carotene</u>- precursor of Vitamin A; acts as antioxidant to potentially help prevent free radical damage.

<u>Beta-glucan</u>- acts as an antioxidant that may help reduce heart disease risk.

<u>Bifidobacterium</u>- healthy bacteria that acts as antioxidant to help promote immunity and may have appetite-suppressant effect on the brain.

<u>Biotin</u>- water soluble vitamin necessary for metabolism of macronutrients and enzyme utilization.

<u>Bisphenol A (BPA)</u>- chemical used in the production of certain plastics.

<u>Body fat percentage</u>- tool used to help determine risk of weight-related diseases.

<u>Body frame size</u>- tool that can be used in conjunction with ideal weight calculation.

Body Mass index- calculation based on height and weight used to measure body fat and future health risks.

Calcium- A mineral necessary for strong bones and teeth.

Cancer- when body cells are destroyed by the production of abnormal cells.

Capsicum- acts an antioxidant to potentially help prevent free radical damage as well as a painkiller.

Carbohydrates- required for body energy, DNA and RNA.

Catechin- antioxidant that may help improve heart health and act as antibacterial.

Chloride- mineral necessary for normal fluid balance.

Cholecystokinin- hormone that signals satiation.

Cholesterol- fatty substance found in cells and an important indicator of heart disease.

Chromium- mineral that helps with metabolism of macronutrients and glucose.

Chronic disease- a disease lasting 3 or more months.

Cobalamin- B12; water soluble vitamin that helps form new blood cells.

Cobalt- mineral that helps prevent anemia.

Complementary protein- the making of a complete protein from combining certain incomplete proteins.

Complete protein- source of protein that provides all of the essential amino acids.

Complex carbohydrate- long chain of mono or disaccharides.

Conjugated linoleic acid- acts as an antioxidant to potentially help maintain body composition and immunity.

Copper- mineral that is required for the absorption and use of iron.

Coronary heart disease- a buildup of plaque in the arteries.

C-reactive protein- indicator of inflammation which can lead to atherosclerosis.

Cushing's syndrome- occurs when the adrenal glands produce too much cortisol.

Diallyl sulfide- an antioxidant that may help detoxify unhealthy compounds.

Dietary fiber- fibers that do not break down within the body.

Disaccharides- double sugars.

Docosahexaenoic acid (DHA)- an omega-3 fatty acid.

Eicosapentaenoic acid (EPA)- an omega-3 fatty acid.

Electrolytes- certain minerals that have an electrical charge.

Empty calories- foods that provide calories but little to no vitamins or minerals.

Energy expenditure- the amount of energy burned through rest, metabolism and activity.

Enriched- nutrients that were lost during processing and were added back to the food or drink.

Essential amino acids- amino acids that must be obtained through foods.

Fasting blood sugar test- blood sugar level test taken after an overnight fast.

Fat- required for cell membranes, carrying fat soluble vitamins, growth and development.

Fat soluble vitamins- vitamins that are absorbed and transported in fats and includes vitamins DEKA.

Flavonol- acts as an antioxidant.

Flavanone- acts as an antioxidant to potentially prevent free radical damage.

Fluoride- mineral that resists acid and decay of teeth.

Folate- water soluble vitamin that helps produce and maintain red blood cells as well as prevent birth defects.

Folic acid- synthetic form of folate.

Fortified- nutrients added to foods or drinks that were not originally in the food or drink.

Free radicals- causes cell and DNA damage through oxidation.

Fructose- single sugars found in fruit.

Functional foods- foods that provide additional health benefits beyond normal nutrition.

Galactose- single sugars found in milk.

Genetically modified organisms- form of biotechnology used to enhance certain traits in crops.

Gherlin- hormone that increases hunger and prompts food intake.

Glucose- blood sugar; single sugars that are the main energy source for cells.

Glycated hemoglobin test (A1C test)- measures average blood sugar levels from past 2-3 months.

Glycemic index- a scale that measures certain foods ability to quickly break down food.

Glycosidic bond- covalent bond where electron pairs are shared between atoms.

Hamwi calculation- a calculation to determine ideal weight.

Heart disease- consists of a myriad of heart problems that can lead to serious injury or death.

Heme iron- iron obtained from animals and better absorbed than plant-based iron.

High biological value protein- synonym for complete protein.

High blood pressure- when pressure against artery walls is higher than normal and can lead to health problems.

High-density lipoprotein- helps lower unhealthy LDL (low-density lipoprotein) levels which has positive health benefits.

Hormones- substances used in animals to enhance growth rate.

Hypothyroidism- when the thyroid does not produce enough thyroid hormone.

Incomplete protein- source of protein that does not provide all of the essential amino acids.

Insoluble fiber- helps with digestive health and acts as antioxidant to potentially reduce cancer risk and reduce appetite.

Inulin- promotes healthy digestive health and acts as an antioxidant to potentially lower risk of cancer, heart disease and obesity.

Iodine- mineral that helps form thyroid hormones.

Iron- mineral that transports oxygen throughout the body for energy production.

Isoflavone- acts as an antioxidant to potentially help bone, immune, and brain health and reduce risk of cancer.

Isomer- when two molecules have the same molecular formula but have different chemical structures.

Jaundice- yellowing of the skin.

Lactobacilli- healthy bacteria that acts as antioxidant to potentially promote immune health as well as appetite-suppressant effect on the brain.

Lactose-double sugars found in milk.

Lean body mass- the amount of body weight that is not fat-related.

Leptin- hormone that helps suppress the appetite and increase energy expenditure.

Lignan- acts as an antioxidant to potentially promote heart and immune health.

Lorcaserin- prescription medication to increase feelings of fullness.

Low biological value protein- synonym for incomplete protein.

Low-density lipoprotein- contributes to atherosclerosis which has negative health effects.

Lutein- antioxidant for potential eye health.

Lycopene- acts as an antioxidant to potentially help prevent DNA and cell damage.

Macronutrients- proteins, fats and carbohydrates that provide calories and energy for the body.

Magnesium- mineral required for genetic material and proper bone growth.

Maltose- double sugars found in malt.

Manganese- mineral required for bone formation.

Medium-chain fatty acid- acts as an antioxidant to potentially help reduce body mass index and fat accumulation.

Metabolic syndrome- a cluster of 3 or more health problems.

Metabolism- chemical reactions that maintain cell life.

Methyl- a carbon atom with 3 hydrogen atoms attached (CH_3).

Micronutrients- vitamins and minerals that are required by the body in small amounts.

Mifflin St. Jeor equation- an equation to determine daily calorie needs.

Molybdenum- mineral that helps with metabolism.

Monosaccharides- single sugars.

Monounsaturated fats- lowers LDL cholesterol and raises HDL cholesterol which has positive health benefits.

MyPlate- a division of U.S. Dept of Agriculture aimed at healthy living .

Neotame- a nonnutritive sweetener.

Niacin- water soluble vitamin that helps enzymes convert food into energy.

Nonessential amino acids- amino acids that they body can make on its own.

Non-heme iron- iron obtained from plants.

Nonnutritive sweeteners- sweeteners that provide lower or zero calories or carbohydrates.

Nutritive sweeteners- sweeteners that provide calories and carbohydrates.

Oligosaccharides- promotes healthy digestive health and acts as an antioxidant to potentially lower risk of cancer, heart disease and obesity.

Omega fatty acids- polyunsaturated fats that must be obtained through foods and are required for brain function and cell growth.

Oral glucose tolerance test- taken after an overnight fast and after drinking a sugary liquid.

Orlistsat- prescription and nonprescription medication that inhibits some fat absorption.

Osteoporosis- when bones become weak and brittle causing an potential increase in bone breakage.

Overweight/obesity- a contributor to 4 of the 6 leading causes of death.

Pantothenic acid- water soluble vitamin needed for energy metabolism.

Peptide YY- hormone that decreases appetite.

Peptide bond- where a carboxyl group (COOH) and amino group (NH₃) interact to form a chemical bond while also releasing water (H₂0).

Pesticides- substances used to prevent damage to crops.

Phentermine- prescription medication to reduce appetite.

Phosphorus- mineral that is required for energy metabolism and growth.

Phytochemical- plant derived components that help protect against disease.

Polysaccharide- large carbohydrate structures that break down to simple sugars.

Polyunsaturated fats- lowers LDL cholesterol which has positive health benefits and has an appetite-reducing effect.

Potassium- mineral that acts as an acid-base balance.

Prebiotic- food for the intestinal bacteria that has positive health benefits.

Proanthocyandins- antioxidant for potential heart and urinary tract health.

Probiotic- bacteria that is found in foods and raises intestinal bacteria counts in a beneficial way.

Processed foods- foods that have been altered from its natural state.

Protein- required for structure, function and chemical reactions within the body.

Pyridoxine- water soluble vitamin that helps absorb protein and carbohydrates.

Quercetin- antioxidant that may help prevent free radical damage.

Random blood sugar test- randomly tested to determine sugar values.

Refined sugars- processed sugars from sugar cane or sugar beet.

Resistant starches- starches that resist digestion in small intestine and act as antioxidant to potentially reduce fat accumulation.

Resveratrol- antioxidant that may slow oxidation and reduce cancer risk.

Riboflavin- water soluble vitamin required for growth and metabolism of foods.

Ribose- part of RNA and DNA.

Rickets- softening and weakening of bones.

Saccharin- Sweet'N Low®; a nonnutritive sweetener.

Satiation- a feeling of fullness and satisfaction.

Saturated fat- raises LDL levels in blood which can lead to health problems.

Scurvy- disease that can cause gum disease and skin hemorrhages.

Selenium- mineral that acts as antioxidant to help prevent free radical damage.

Self-efficacy- the belief you have in yourself in order to follow through to success.

Set point theory- the body's desire to maintain a certain weight and fat content.

Simple carbohydrate- simple sugars found naturally in fruits and milk.

Small-chain fatty acids- may have appetite-suppressant effect on brain.

SMART rules- a guide to goal setting.

Sodium- mineral that helps regulate fluid and blood volume.

Soluble fiber- may help reduce heart disease and act as antioxidant to potentially reduce cancer risk and obesity.

Soy protein- acts as an antioxidant to potentially help reduce risk of heart disease.

Stanol- antioxidant that may help reduce risk of heart disease.

Starch- a polysaccharide.

Sterol- antioxidant that may help reduce risk of heart disease.

Steriochemistry- the arrangement of atoms to form a molecular structure.

Stevia- an artificial sweetener.

Stroke- a condition that occurs when blood flow to the brain becomes blocked.

Sucralose- Splenda®; a nonnutritive sweetener.

Sucrose- double sugars found in table sugar.

Sugar alcohol- acts as an antioxidant to help prevent cavities.

Sulforaphane- antioxidant that may help detoxify unhealthy compounds.

Sulfur- mineral that is an essential part of amino acids.

Target heart rate- calculation used to determine optimal exercise rate.

Thiamine- water soluble vitamin necessary for carbohydrate metabolism.

Thyroid test- measures thyroid stimulating hormone in blood.

Trans fat- raises LDL cholesterol and lowers HDL cholesterol which can lead to health problems.

Triglyceride- the storage form of fat.

Type 1 diabetes- genetic disease where the body produces too little insulin to properly regulate blood glucose.

Type 2 diabetes- develops when the body is unable to utilize insulin properly for blood glucose control.

Vegetarians- those that do not eat meat, fish or poultry.

Vitamin A- fat soluble vitamin essential for eyesight and acts as an antioxidant for potential protection from free radicals.

Vitamin D- fat soluble vitamin that helps calcium absorption.

Vitamin E- fat soluble vitamin that helps form red blood cells, muscles and other tissues and acts as an antioxidant for potential protection from free radicals.

Vitamin K- fat soluble vitamin that assists in blood clotting.

Waist Circumference- a tool to determine possible future health risks.

Water soluble vitamins- vitamins that are absorbed and transported in water and includes B vitamins and Vitamin C.

Weight management- the development of healthy eating and physical activity habits in support of lifelong well-being and healthy weight.

Zinc- mineral that helps form protein and required for growth and development.

Resources:

1. Healthy Reflections. Cornell University website. http://foodpsychology.cornell.edu/JACR/Healthy_Reflections. Updated 2016. Accessed January 15, 2016.

2. Mahan K, Raymond J, Stump S. Chapter 2: Estimating Energy Requirements: Mifflin St. Jeor. In: Mahan K, Raymond J, Stump S, eds. *Krause's Food and the Nutrition Care Process.* 13th ed. St. Louis, Missouri: Elsevier; 2012: 24.

3. Walker G. ed. Chapter 2: Body Mass Index. In: Walker G, ed. *Pocket Resource for Nutrition Assessement. Consultant Dietetians In Health Care Facilities.* 7th ed. 2009: 25-29.

4. Assessing Your Weight. Centers for Disease Control and Prevention. http://www.cdc.gov/healthyweight/assessing. Updated May 15, 2015. Accessed January 15, 2016.

5. Walker G. ed. Chapter 2 : Ideal Body Weight (IBW). In: Walker G, ed. *Pocket Resource for Nutrition Assessement. Consultant Dietetians In Health Care Facilities.* 7th ed. City, State, Publisher, 2009: 19-22.

6. Other Factors in Weight Gain. Centers for Disease Control and Prevention website. http://www.cdc.gov/healthyweight/calories/other_factors.html. Updated May 15, 2016. Accessed January 21, 2016.

7. Hensrud, D. Weight Loss: Better to Cut Calories or Exercise More? Mayo Clinic website. http://www.mayoclinic.org/healthy-lifestyle/weight-loss/expert-answers/weight-loss/faq-20058292. March 4, 2014. Accessed January 23, 2016

8. Walk, Don't Run, Your Way to a Healthy Heart. American Heart Association website. https://www.heart.org/HEARTORG/HealthyLiving/PhysicalActivity/Walking/Walk-Dont-Run-Your-Way-to-a-Healthy-Heart_UCM_452926_Article.jsp?appName=MobileApp. Updated March 2014. Accessed January 23, 2016

9. What Causes Overweight and Obesity? National Institutes of Health website. http://www.nhlbi.nih.gov/health/health-topics/topics/obe/causes. Updated July 13, 2012. Accessed January 21, 2016.

10. How to Change Emotional Eating. WebMD website. http://www.webmd.com/parenting/raising-fit-kids/mood/change-emotional-eating. Updated February 25, 2015. Accessed January 21, 2016

11. Physical Activity Reduces Stress. Anxiety and Depression Association of America website. http://www.adaa.org/understanding-anxiety/related-illnesses/other-related-conditions/stress/physical-activity-reduces-st. Updated 2016. Accessed January 22, 2016

12. Kyle T, Kuehl, B. Prescription Medications and Weight Gain: What You Need to Know. Obesity Action Coalition website. http://www.obesityaction.org/educational-resources/resource-articles-2/general-articles/prescription-medications-weight-gain. 2016. Accessed January 22, 2016.

13. What Causes Overweight and Obesity? National Institutes of Health website. http://www.nhlbi.nih.gov/health/health-topics/topics/obe/causes. July 13, 2012. Accessed January 22, 2016.

14. General Information/Press Room. American Thyroid Association website. http://www.thyroid.org/media-main/about-hypothyroidism/. 2016. Accessed January 22, 2016

15. What Causes Overweight and Obesity? National Institutes of Health website. http://www.nhlbi.nih.gov/health/health-topics/topics/obe/causes. July 13, 2012. Accessed January 24, 2016.

16. Set-Point Theory. The Center for Health Promotion and Wellness. MIT Medical website. https://medical.mit.edu/sites/default/files/set_point_theory.pdf. Accessed January 24, 2016

17. Weight Management: Strategies for Success. Nutrition.gov website. http://www.nutrition.gov/weight-management/strategies-success/interested-losing-weight. Accessed January 24, 2016

18. Weight Loss: Strategies for Success. Mayo Clinic website. http://www.mayoclinic.org/healthy-lifestyle/weight-loss/in-depth/weight-loss/art-20047752. Updated November 16, 2015. Accessed January 24, 2016.

19. 5 Steps to Lose Weight. American Heart Association website. http://www.heart.org/HEARTORG/GettingHealthy/WeightManagement/LosingWeight/5-Steps-to-Lose-Weight_UCM_307260_Article.jsp#.VpkjTFKbUZw. January 13, 2016. Accessed January 25, 2016

20. Bauer K, Liou D, Sokolik C. Chapter 4: Nutritional Counseling Motivational Algorithm. In: Bauer K, Liou D, Sokolik C, eds. *Nutrition Counseling and Education Skill Development.* 3rd ed. Boston, MA: Cengage; 2012: 79.

21. Dodson F. Quote.
http://www.sparkpeople.com/resource/quotes_translation.asp?id=111. Accessed January 25, 2016.

22. Set Your Weight Loss Goals. United States Department of Veterans Affairs website. http://www.move.va.gov/docs/NewHandouts/Standard/S02_SetYourWeightLossGoals .pdf. Accessed January 25, 2016

23. Chronic Diseases: The Leading Causes of Death and Disability in the United States. Centers for Disease Control and Prevention website. http://www.cdc.gov/chronicdisease/overview/. Updated February 23, 2015. Accessed January 29, 2016

24. About Metabolic Syndrome. American Heart Association website. http://www.heart.org/HEARTORG/Conditions/More/MetabolicSyndrome/About-Metabolic-Syndrome_UCM_301920_Article.jsp#.Vt2eB-abUlA. Updated May 14, 2014. Accessed January 29, 2016.

25. Unhealthy Eating and Physical Inactivity Cause 1/3 of Premature Deaths. National Alliance for Nutrition and Activity website. https://cspinet.org/new/pdf/cdc_briefing_book_fy10.pdf /. 2010. Accessed January 29, 2016.

26. Mahan K, Raymond J, Stump S. Chapter 37: Medical Nutrition Therapy for Cancer Prevention, Treatment and Recover. In: Mahan K, Raymond J, Stump S, ed. *Krause's Food and the Nutrition Care Process*. 13th Edition. St. Louis, Missouri: Elsevier; 2012: 833.

27. American Cancer Society Guidelines on Nutrition and Physical Activity for Cancer Prevention. American Cancer Society website. http://www.cancer.org/acs/groups/cid/documents/webcontent/002577-pdf.pdf. Updated February 5, 2015. Accessed January 29, 2016.

28. What Causes a Stroke? National Institutes of Health website. https://www.nhlbi.nih.gov/health/health-topics/topics/stroke/causes. Updated October 28, 2015. Accessed January 30, 2016.

29. Your Guide to Diabetes: Type 1 and Type 2. U.S. Department of Health and Human Services website. http://www.niddk.nih.gov/health-information/health-topics/Diabetes/your-guide-diabetes/Pages/index.aspx. Updated February 2014. Accessed January 30, 2016

30. Simple Steps to Preventing Diabetes. Harvard School of Public Health website. http://www.hsph.harvard.edu/nutritionsource/preventing-diabetes-full-story/. Accessed February 2, 2016.

31. Losing Weight: What is Healthy Weight Loss? Centers for Disease Control and Prevention websitehttp://www.cdc.gov/healthyweight/losing_weight/. Updated February 2, 2015. Accessed March 29, 2016.

32. Alberts B, Johnson A, Lewis J., et al. Chapter 3: . In: Alberts B, Johnson A, Lewis J, eds. *Molecular Biology of the Cell.* 4th ed. New York: Garland Science; 2002: 129

33. Shaw D, Canagaratnam M. Chapter 2: Explanation: Dietary Aspects of Amino Acids. In Shaw D, Canagaratnam M, eds. *Metabolism and Nutrition.* Boca Rotan, FL: CRC Press; 2005: 53.

34. Protein. Harvard School of Public Health website. http://www.hsph.harvard.edu/nutritionsource/what-should-you-eat/protein/. Accessed February 2, 2016.

35. Seagar S, Slabaugh M. Chapter 9: Can a Higher Protein Diet Help Me Lose Weight? In: Seagar s, Slabaugh M, eds. *Organic and Biochemistry for Today.* 8th ed. Belmont, CA: Cengage; 2014: 271

36. Protein. Utah Department of Health website. http://health.utah.gov/wic/pdf/forms_and_modules/Staff_Training_Modules/Basic%20Nutrition/basic%20nutrition%20module%205.11_files/Page322.htm. Updated May 2011. Accessed February 2, 2016.

37. Eggs and Heart Disease. School of Public Health website. http://www.hsph.harvard.edu/nutritionsource/eggs/. Accessed February 2, 2016.

38. Guzman S. What are Complementary Proteins and How Do we Get Them? Bastyr University website. http://bastyr.edu/news/health-tips/2011/09/what-are-complementary-proteins-and-how-do-we-get-them. May 1, 2011. Accessed February 9, 2016.

39. Carbohydrates. U.S. National Library of Medicine website. https://www.nlm.nih.gov/medlineplus/ency/article/002469.htm. February 9, 2016. Accessed February 9, 2016.

40. Carbohydrates. Royal Society of Chemistry website. http://www.rsc.org/Education/Teachers/Resources/cfb/carbohydrates.htm. November 2004. Accessed February 9, 2016.

41. Carbohydrate Food Intake and Energy Balance. Food and Agriculture Organization website. http://www.fao.org/docrep/w8079e/w8079e0m.htm. Accessed February 9, 2016.

42. The Carbohydrates: Sugar, Starch and Fiber. Mississippi College powepoint. https://www.mc.edu/faculty/index.php/download_file/8104/7/ Accessed February 29, 2016.

43. How to Use the Glycemic Index. WebMD website. http://www.webmd.com/diabetes/guide/glycemic-index-good-versus-bad-carbs. Accessed Updated June 2014. February 9, 2016.

44. Davis J. Top 10 Sources of Fiber. WebMD website. http://www.webmd.com/diet/features/top-10-sources-of-fiber. October 7, 2005. Accessed February 10, 2016.

45. Fats 101. American Heart Association website. http://www.heart.org/HEARTORG/HealthyLiving/FatsAndOils/Fats-101_UCM_304494_Article.jsp#.Vqjt31KbUZw. Updated February 29, 2016. Accessed February 10, 2016.

46. Good vs. Bad Cholesterol. American Heart Association website. http://www.heart.org/HEARTORG/Conditions/Cholesterol/AboutCholesterol/Good-vs-Bad-Cholesterol_UCM_305561_Article.jsp#.Vqj0t1KbUZw. Updated March 23, 2016. Accessed February 10, 2016.

47. Schmitz G Grandl M. The Molecular Mechanisms of HDL and Associated Vesicular Trafficking Mechanisms to Mediate Cellular Lipid Homeostasis. *ATVBAHA*.2009; 108.179507. http://dx.doi.org/10.1161/ATVBAHA.108.179507.

48. Trans fat is Double Trouble for Your Heart Health. Mayo Clinic website. http://www.mayoclinic.org/diseases-conditions/high-blood-cholesterol/in-depth/trans-fat/art-20046114. Updated June 19, 2015. Accessed February 10, 2016.

49. Christensen J. FDA Orders Food Manufacturers to Stop Using Trans Fat Within Three Years. *CNN Health*. http://www.cnn.com/2015/06/16/health/fda-trans-fat/. June 16, 2015. Accessed February 10, 2016.

50. Hongu N, Wise J, Poschman K. Healthy Fats: Guide for Improving the Quality of Fat Intake. The University of Alabama website. https://extension.arizona.edu/sites/extension.arizona.edu/files/pubs/az1452-2014.pdf. June 2014. Accessed February 10, 2016.

51. Facts about Polyunsaturated Fats. U.S. National Library of Medicine website. https://www.nlm.nih.gov/medlineplus/ency/patientinstructions/000747.htm. Updated May 18, 2014. Accessed February 10, 2016.

52. Aluko R. Chapter 2: Omega-3 and Omega-6 Fatty Acids. In: Aluko R, ed. *Functional Food and Nutraceuticals*. New York, NY: Springer; 2012: 24-28.

53. Simopoulos A. The Importance of the Ratio of Omega-3/Omega-6 Essential Fatty Acids. *Biomed Pharmacother*. 2002 Oct; 56(8): 365-79. https://www.ncbi.nlm.nih.gov/pubmed/12442909. Accessed. February 13, 2016.

54. Dietary References Intake: Macronutients. National Academies of Sciences website. http://www.nationalacademies.org/hmd/~/media/Files/Activity%20Files/Nutrition/DRIs/DRI_Macronutrients.pdf. Updated 2009. Accessed February 15, 2016.

55. Macronutrients: The Importance of Carbohydrate, Protein and Fat. McKinley Health Center website. http://www.mckinley.illinois.edu/handouts/macronutrients.htm. Updated 2014. Accessed February 15, 2016.

56. Brown, J. Chapter 1: Water. In: Brown J, ed. *Nutrition Through The Life Cycle*. 5th ed. Stanford, CT: Cengage; 2014: 24.

57. Water and Nutrition. Centers for Disease Control and Prevention website. http://www.cdc.gov/healthywater/drinking/nutrition/. Updated June 3, 2014. Accessed February 15, 2016.

58. Dietary Reference Intakes: Electrolytes and Water. National Academies of Sciences website. http://iom.nationalacademies.org/Global/News%20Announcements/~/media/442A08B899F44DF9AAD083D86164C75B.ashx. Accessed February 15, 2016.

59. Brown, J. Chapter 1: Water. In: Brown J, ed. *Nutrition Through The Life Cycle*. 5th ed. Stanford, CT: Cengage; 2014: 24.

60. Mahan K, Raymond J, Stump S. Chapter 2: Estimating Energy Requirements: Mifflin St. Jeor. In: Mahan K, Raymond J, Stump S, eds. *Krause's Food and the Nutrition Care Process*. 13th ed. St. Louis, Missouri: Elsevier; 2012: 1142.

61. Walker G, ed. Chapter 2: Body Mass Index. In: Walker G, ed. *Pocket Resource for Nutrition Assessement. Consultant Dietetians In Health Care Facilities*; 7th ed., 2005: 54.

62. Micronutrient Facts. Centers for Disease Control and Prevention website. http://www.cdc.gov/immpact/micronutrients/. Updated March 31, 2015. Accessed February 15, 2016.

63. Argen S. Basic Vitamins: Water-Soluble and Fat- Soluble. University of California at Berkley website. http://www.uen.org/Lessonplan/preview.cgi?LPid=1261. July 9, 1997. Accessed: February 18, 2016.

64. Zelman K. Know the Difference Between Fat and Water Soluble Nutrients. WebMD website. http://www.webmd.com/vitamins-and-supplements/nutrition-vitamins-11/fat-water-nutrient. Updated August 28, 2011. Accessed: February 18, 2016.

65. Calcium and Vitamin D: Important at Every Age. National Institutes of Health website. http://www.niams.nih.gov/Health_Info/Bone/Bone_Health/Nutrition/. Updated May 2015. Accessed February 19, 2016.

66. Why Should I Limit Sodium? American Heart Association website. https://www.heart.org/idc/groups/heart-public/@wcm/@hcm/documents/downloadable/ucm_300625.pdf. Updated 2015. Accessed February 19, 2016.

67. Electrolytes. U.S. National Library of Medicine website. https://www.nlm.nih.gov/medlineplus/ency/article/002350.htm. Updated August 3, 2013. Accessed February 19, 2016.

68. Nutrition and Health Eating. Mayo Clinic website. http://www.mayoclinic.org/healthy-lifestyle/nutrition-and-healthy-eating/in-depth/vegetarian-diet/art-20046446?pg=2. Updated March 14, 2016. Accessed February 19, 2016.

69. Antioxidants and Cancer Prevention. National Institutes of Health website. http://www.cancer.gov/about-cancer/causes-prevention/risk/diet/antioxidants-fact-sheet. Updated January 16, 2014. Accessed February 22, 2016.

70. Are Health Claims of Functional and Fortified Foods True? Academy of Nutrition and Dietetics website. http://www.eatright.org/resource/food/nutrition/healthy-eating/functional-foods. Updated January 31, 2014. Accessed February 22, 2016.

71. Heneman K, Zidenberg-Cherr S. Some Facts About Phytochemicals. University of California website. http://cetulare.ucanr.edu/files/32436.pdf. Updated October 2008. Accessed February 22, 2016.

72. Antioxidants and Cancer Prevention. National Cancer Institute website. https://www.cancer.gov/about-cancer/causes-prevention/risk/diet/antioxidants-fact-sheet. Updated January 2014. Accessed February 22, 2016.

73. Antioxidants. U.S. National Library of Medicine website. https://www.nlm.nih.gov/medlineplus/antioxidants.html. Updated April 2, 2015. Accessed February 22, 2016.

74. Functional Foods Fact Sheet: Antioxidants. International Food Information Council Foundation website. http://www.foodinsight.org/Functional_Foods_Fact_Sheet_Antioxidants. Updated February 20, 2015. Accessed February 22, 2016.

75. Aluko R. In: Aluko R, ed. *Functional Food and Nutraceuticals*. New York, NY: Springer; 2012.

76. Alcohol: Balancing Risks and Benefits. Harvard School of Public Health website. http://www.hsph.harvard.edu/nutritionsource/alcohol-full-story/. Accessed February 22, 2016.

77. Horrocks L, Yeo Y. Health Benefits of Docosahexaenoic Acid (DHA). *Pharmacol Res*. 1999 Sep;40(3):211-25. Doi: 10.1006/phrs.1999.0495.

78. Processed Foods: What's OK, What to Avoid. Academy of Nutrition and Dietetics website. http://www.eatright.org/resource/food/nutrition/nutrition-facts-and-food-labels/avoiding-processed-foods. Updated November 9, 2015. Accessed February 22, 2016.

79. Natural vs. Refined Sugars: What's the Difference? Cancer Treatment Centers of America website. http://www.cancercenter.com/discussions/blog/natural-vs-refined-sugars-whats-the-difference/. Updated July 30, 2014. Accessed February 24, 2016.

80. What You Need to Know About Preservatives. EatRight Ontario website. http://www.eatrightontario.ca/en/Articles/Food-technology/Biotechnology/Novel-foods/What-you-need-to-know-about-preservatives.aspx#.VrIc91KbUZw. Updated 2016. Accessed February 24, 2016.

81. Generally Recognized as Safe (GRAS). U.S. Food and Drug Administration website. http://www.fda.gov/Food/IngredientsPackagingLabeling/GRAS/. Updated June 4, 2015. Accessed February 24, 2016.

82. Pesticides: What are Pesticides? U.S. National Library of Medicine website. http://toxtown.nlm.nih.gov/text_version/chemicals.php?id=23. Updated December 15, 2015. Accessed February 29, 2016.

83. Understanding Food Marketing Terms. Academy of Nutrition and Dietetics website. http://www.eatright.org/resource/food/nutrition/nutrition-facts-and-food-labels/understanding-food-marketing-terms. Updated February 5, 2014. Accessed Feburary 29, 2016.

84. Steroid Hormone Implants Used for Growth in Food-Producing Animals. U.S. Food and Drug Administration website. http://www.fda.gov/AnimalVeterinary/SafetyHealth/ProductSafetyInformation/ucm055436.htm. Updated October 20, 2015. Accessed February 29, 2016.

85. Phasing Out Certain Antibiotic Use in Farm Animals. U.S. Food and Drug Administration website. http://www.fda.gov/ForConsumers/ConsumerUpdates/ucm378100.htm. Updated December 11, 2013. Accessed February 29, 2016.

86. Understanding Food Marketing Terms. Academy of Nutrition and Dietetics website. http://www.eatright.org/resource/food/nutrition/nutrition-facts-and-food-labels/understanding-food-marketing-terms. Updated February 4, 2014.Accessed March 1, 2016.

87. Plastics that May be Harmful to Children and Reproductive Health. Environment and Human Health, Inc. website. http://www.ehhi.org/reports/plastics/bpa_health_effects.shtml. Updated. Accessed March 1, 2016.

88. Bisphenol A (BPA): Use in Food Contact Application. U.S. Food and Drug Administration website. http://www.fda.gov/NewsEvents/PublicHealthFocus/ucm064437.htm. Updated November 2014. Accessed March 1, 2016.

89. Bisphenol A (BPA). National Institutes of Health website. http://www.niehs.nih.gov/health/topics/agents/sya-bpa/. Accessed March 1, 2016.

90. A Science-Based Look at Genetically Engineered Crops. The National Academies of Sciences website. http://nas-sites.org/ge-crops/. Updated 2014. Accessed March 1, 2016.

91. The Impact of Genetically Engineered Crops on Farm Sustainability in the United States. National Academies of Sciences website. http://www.nationalacademies.org/includes/genengcrops.pdf. Updated 2010. Accessed March 1, 2016.

92. Genetically Modified Foods. Food and Nutrition Conference and Expo website. http://fnce.eatright.org/fnce/uploaded/635200401044706971-453.%20Malamy.pdf. Updated November 13, 2013. Accessed March 1, 2016.

93. Fitch C, Keim K. Position of the Academy of Nutrition and Dietetics: Use of Nutritive and Nonnutritive Sweeteners. *J Acad Nutr Diet*. 2012; 112: 739-758. http://www.eatrightpro.org/resource/practice/position-and-practice-papers/position-papers/use-of-nutritive-and-nonnutritive-sweeteners. Accessed March 1, 2016.

94. Additional Information about High-Intensity Sweeteners Permitted for use in Food in the United States. U.S. Food and Drug Administration website. http://www.fda.gov/Food/IngredientsPackagingLabeling/FoodAdditivesIngredients/ucm397725.htm /. Updated May 25, 2016. Accessed March 1, 2016.

95. Is Stevia an 'FDA Approved' Sweetener? U.S. Food and Drug Administration website. http://www.fda.gov/AboutFDA/Transparency/Basics/ucm214864.htm. Updated March 25, 2016. Accessed March 30, 2016.

96. Artificial Sweeteners and Cancer. National Institutes Health website. http://www.cancer.gov/about-cancer/causes-prevention/risk/diet/artificial-sweeteners-fact-sheet. Updated August 5, 2009. Accessed March 3, 2016.

97. Kyle T, Hignett W. Ghrelin, the "Go" Hormone. Obesity Action Coalition. http://www.obesityaction.org/educational-resources/resource-articles-2/general-articles/ghrelin-the-go-hormone. Accessed March 0, 2016.

98. Cauter E, Knutson K, Leproult R, Spiegel K. The Impact of Sleep Deprivation on Hormones and Metabolism. *Sleep Med*. 2008 Sep; 9 (01): S23-S28. Doi: 10.1016/S1389-9457(08)70013-3.

99. Graaf C, Blom W, Smeets P, Stafleu A, Hendriks H. Biomarkers of Satiation and Satiety. *Am J Clin Nutr*. 2004 June; 79(6): 946-961. http://ajcn.nutrition.org/content/79/6/946.long. Accessed March 5, 2016.

100. Klok, M, Jakobsdottir, S, Drent, M. The Role of Leptin and Ghrelin in the Regulation of Food Intake and Body Weight in Humans: a Review. *Obesity Reviews*, 8: 21–34. Doi: 10.1111/j.1467-789X.2006.00270.x.

101. Karra E, Chandarana K, Batterham R. The Role of Peptide YY in Appetite Regulation and Obesity. *J Physiol*. 2009 Jan; 587 (Pt 1): 19-25. Doi: 10.1113/jphysiol.2008.164269.

102. Weight Loss. Mayo Clinic website. http://www.mayoclinic.org/healthy-lifestyle/weight-loss/in-depth/weight-loss-drugs/art-20044832?pg=2. Updated April 30, 2015. Accessed March 30, 2016.

103. Hensrud D. Alli Weight-Loss Pill: Does it Work? Mayo Clinic website. http://www.mayoclinic.org/healthy-lifestyle/weight-loss/in-depth/alli/art-20047908. February 7, 2015. Accessed March 3, 2016.

104. Recommendations for Physical Activity. National Institutes of Health website. https://www.nhlbi.nih.gov/health/health-topics/topics/phys/recommend. Updated October 29, 2015. Accessed March 3, 2016.

105. Potential Benefits of Regular Moderate Physical Activity. Cengage. http://www.cengage.com/resource_uploads/downloads/0840064152_296702.pdf. Accessed March 5, 2016.

106. Keeping it Off. Centers for Disease Control and Prevention website. http://www.cdc.gov/healthyweight/losing_weight/keepingitoff.html. Updated May 15, 2015. Accessed March 5, 2016.

107. Robinson K. Circuit Training. WebMD website. http://www.webmd.com/fitness-exercise/a-z/circuit-training. 2014. Accessed March 5, 2016.

108. Weight Loss: How Much am I Burning? Mayo Clinic website. http://www.mayoclinic.org/healthy-lifestyle/weight-loss/in-depth/exercise/art-20050999?pg=2. Updated November 15, 2014. Accessed March 5, 2016.

109. Target Heart Rates. American Heart Association website. http://www.heart.org/HEARTORG/HealthyLiving/PhysicalActivity/FitnessBasics/Target-Heart-Rates_UCM_434341_Article.jsp#.Vt-FZ-abUlA. Updated January 13, 2016. Accessed March 5, 2016.

110. Behavioral Change Models: The Health Belief Model. Boston University School of Public Health website. http://sphweb.bumc.bu.edu/otlt/MPH-Modules/SB/SB721-Models/SB721-Models2.html /. Updated January 6, 2016. Accessed March 6, 2016.

111. Carey M, Forsyth A. Teaching Tip Sheet: Self-Efficacy. American Psychological Association website. http://www.apa.org/pi/aids/resources/education/self-efficacy.aspx. Accessed March 30, 2016.

112. Bouchez C. Can Stress Cause Weight Gain? WebMD website. http://www.webmd.com/diet/can-stress-cause-weight-gain. 2005. Accessed March 6, 2016.

113. Ramanujan K. Keeping Track of Weight Daily May Tip Scale in Your Favor. Cornell University website. http://news.cornell.edu/stories/2015/06/keeping-track-weight-daily-may-tip-scale-your-favor. June 12, 2015. Accessed March 6, 2016.

114. Social Support: A Necessity for Weight Loss. Mayo Clinic website. http://diet.mayoclinic.org/diet/motivate/social-support-for-weight-loss?xid=nl_MayoClinicDiet_20151021. Accessed March 6, 2016.

Table Resources

Table 1: Serving-Size Chart. Dairy Council of California website.
http://www.healthyeating.org/Portals/0/Documents/Tip%20Sheets/Portion_Serving_ Size_Chart_Eng.pdf. Accessed January 9, 2016.

Table 2: Estimated Calorie Needs per Day by Age, Gender, and Physical Activity Level. Center for Nutrition Policy and Promotion, USDA.
http://www.cnpp.usda.gov/sites/default/files/usda_food_patterns/EstimatedCalorieNe edsPerDayTable.pdf. Accessed January 9, 2016.

Table 3: USDA Food Patterns. Center for Nutrition Policy and Promotion, USDA.
http://www.cnpp.usda.gov/sites/default/files/usda_food_patterns/USDAFoodPatterns SummaryTable.pdf. Accessed January 9, 2016.

Table 4: USDA Food Patterns. Center for Nutrition Policy and Promotion, USDA.
http://www.cnpp.usda.gov/sites/default/files/usda_food_patterns/USDAFoodPatterns SummaryTable.pdf. Accessed January 12, 2016.

Table 5: Body Mass Index Table. National Institutes of Health.
http://www.nhlbi.nih.gov/health/educational/lose_wt/BMI/bmi_tbl.pdf. Accessed March 30, 2016.

Table 6: Calculating Body Frame Size. U.S. National Library of Medicine. August 17, 2014.
https://www.nlm.nih.gov/medlineplus/ency/imagepages/17182.htm. Accessed March 30, 2016.

Table 7: Bauer K, Liou D, Sokolik C. Chapter 4: Nutritional Counseling Motivational Algorithm. In: Bauer K, Liou D, Sokolik C, eds. *Nutrition Counseling and Education Skill Development*. Boston, MA: Cengage; 3rd ed. 2012: 413.

Table 8: Blood Tests For Heart Disease. Mayo Clinic website.
http://www.mayoclinic.org/diseases-conditions/heart-disease/in-depth/heart-disease/art-20049357. Updated June 5, 2014. Accessed January 12, 2016.

Table 9: Diabetes: Tests and Diagnosis. Mayo Clinic website.
http://www.mayoclinic.org/diseases-conditions/diabetes/basics/tests-diagnosis/con-20033091. Updated July 31, 2014. Accessed January 12, 2016.

Table 10: Obesity: Tests and Diagnosis. Mayo Clinic website.
http://www.mayoclinic.org/diseases-conditions/obesity/basics/tests-diagnosis/con-20014834. Updated June 10, 2015. Accessed January 24, 2016.

Table 11: Protein Content of Foods. Today's Dietitian website.

http://www.todaysdietitian.com/pdf/webinars/ProteinContentofFoods.pdf. Accessed March 30, 2016.

Table 12: Soy for Heart Disease. Soyfoods Association of North America website. http://www.soyfoods.org/nutrition-health/soy-for-healthy-living/soy-for-heart-disease/soy-protein-content-chart. Accessed January 24, 2016. and

Table 12: Mangels R. Protein in the Vegan Diet. The Vegetarian Resource Group website. https://www.vrg.org/nutrition/protein.php. Updated 2016. Accessed March 30, 2016.

Table 13: Protein Content of Foods. Today's Dietitian website. http://www.todaysdietitian.com/pdf/webinars/ProteinContentofFoods.pdf. Accessed March 30, 2016.

Table 14-19: Brown J. Chapter 1: Carbohydrates. In: Brown J, ed. *Nutrition Through The Life Cycle*. 5th ed. Stanford, CT: Cengage; 2014: 5-7.

Table 20: Estimated Calorie Needs per Day by Age, Gender, and Physical Activity Level. Center for Nutrition Policy and Promotion, USDA website. http://www.cnpp.usda.gov/sites/default/files/usda_food_patterns/EstimatedCalorieNeedsPerDayTable.pdf. Accessed Feb 2, 2016

Table 21-50: Learning about Vitamins and Minerals. Food and Agriculture Organization website. http://www.fao.org/docrep/017/i3261e/i3261e06.pdf. Accessed March 30, 2016. And Nutrient Chart: Function, Deficiency, and Toxicity Symptoms, and Major Food Sources. WICWorks Resource System website. https://wicworks.fns.usda.gov/wicworks//Topics/FG/AppendixC_NutrientChart.pdf. Accessed February 2, 2016.

Table 51-62: Aluko R. Chapter 2: Omega-3 and Omega-6 Fatty Acids. In: Aluko R, ed. *Functional Food and Nutraceuticals*. New York, NY: Springer; 2012. And Functional Foods Fact Sheet: Antioxidants. FoodInsight.org. http://www.foodinsight.org/ Functional _Foods_Fact_Sheet_Antioxidants. Accessed January 25, 2017.

Table 63: Calories Burned in 30 Minutes for People of Three Different Weights. Harvard Health Publications website. http://www.health.harvard.edu/diet-and-weight-loss/calories-burned-in-30-minutes-of-leisure-and-routine-activities. Updated January 27, 2016. Accessed February 2, 2016.

Table 64: Target Heart Rates. American Heart Association website. http://www.heart.org/HEARTORG/HealthyLiving/PhysicalActivity/FitnessBasics/Target-Heart-Rates_UCM_434341_Article.jsp#.VrtieVKbUlA. Updated January 2015. Accessed February 2, 2016.

Table 65: What are the Guidelines for Percentage of Body Fat Loss? ACE Fitness website. http://www.acefitness.org/acefit/healthy-living-article/60/112/what-are-the-guidelines-for-percentage-of/. Updated December 2, 2009. Accessed March 6, 2016.

www.ingramcontent.com/pod-product-compliance
Lightning Source LLC
Chambersburg PA
CBHW081346280526
45788CB00009B/2793